PICTURE PERFECT WEIGHT LOSS 30-DAY PLAN

Dr Howard M. Shapiro

RODALE

This edition first published in 2005 by
Rodale International Ltd
7–10 Chandos Street
London W1G 9AD
www.rodale.co.uk

Printed and bound by Shenzhen Donnelley Bright Sun Printing Co., Ltd
1 3 5 7 9 8 6 4 2

A CIP record for this book is available from the British Library
ISBN 1-4050-7739-5

This paperback edition distributed to the book trade by Pan Macmillan Ltd

Produced for Rodale International Ltd by
studio cactus Ⓒ
Designed by Dawn Terrey
Edited by Aaron Brown

Cover photography by Iain Bagwell (see pages 148-9 for calorie equations).
Interior photographs by Iain Bagwell except: Kurt Wilson/Rodale images: 8, 58 (sliced bread),
59 (sliced bread), 92, 93 (cheese), 99, 102 (crisps), 104, 108, 109, 116, 126, 127, 134, 136, 140, 154,
159, 162, 165. Photos.com: pages 6, 10, 12, 21, 23, 24, 30, 32, 34, 36, 41, 44, 46, 49, 51, 52, 55,
56, 67, 69, 72, 73, 86, 87, 88, 89, 110, 112, 128, 144, 146. PhotoDisc: pages 11, 38, 48.
Stockbyte: page 27. Studio Cactus: pages 15, 28, 29, 35, 58 (French bread), 60, 61, 62, 63,
81 (bananas), 102 (breadsticks), 106, 107.

www.drhowardshapiro.com

Notice

This book is intended as a reference volume only, not as a medical manual. The information given
here is designed to help you make informed decisions about your health. It is not intended as a
substitute for any treatment that may have been prescribed by your doctor. If you suspect that you
have a medical problem, we urge you to seek competent medical help.

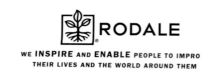

WE **INSPIRE** AND **ENABLE** PEOPLE TO IMPRO
THEIR LIVES AND THE WORLD AROUND THEM

To Kay von Bergen
With deep appreciation and great respect.
Simply put, thank you . . .

In memory of Paul Pansini and Raymond Meisenheimer
and in honour of their brethren, New York City's firefighters –
'The Bravest' – who responded to the tragedy of
September 11, 2001 with uncommon valour,
reclaiming for us all a sense of human decency
and exemplifying the true meaning of heroism.

CONTENTS

CHAPTER 1: WEIGHT LOSS & REAL LIFE – *YOUR* REAL LIFE

You're reading this book because you're overweight – or perhaps someone in your family is overweight – and you're unhappy about it. But you can put an end to this situation. Right now.

For more than 25 years I've treated patients who claim they have 'tried everything' and been unable to lose weight. I've treated those who put back on all the weight they had lost

> ## Weight gain is happening everywhere around the world

on popular diet programmes. I've worked with patients who have followed every fad from hypnosis to fasting; patients who have measured portions and counted every gram of fat; patients who have deprived themselves of foods they love, forced themselves to eat foods they don't particularly like, eaten meals when a book or diet guru told them to, and beaten themselves up every time they had a biscuit or asked for a second helping.

WHO DIETS?

I've worked with everyone: children and the elderly, high-powered executives, celebrities, politicians, full-time mothers, people who eat on the run and people who regularly dine at the world's finest restaurants. I've helped them understand why diets don't work, why deprivation is counter-productive, why fasting can actually harm you. I've taught them what this book will teach you in 30 days: that there is a way of eating – eating the

foods you enjoy eating and eating them until you feel satisfied – that actually helps you lose weight and keep it off. I call it Picture Perfect Weight Loss. Yes, that's partly because you can see the difference in yourself as you lose weight. But mostly, Picture Perfect Weight Loss refers to the method I use in my practice for teaching this way of eating. The nutritionists on my staff continually create food comparison demonstrations that show patients a range of food options and allow them to compare the weight-loss consequences of each. As you'll see, we've reproduced our food demos in the photographs in this book. They provide vivid lessons in how you can eat healthy, delicious food for the rest of your life and still lose weight and keep it off.

How can I be so sure? Because Picture Perfect Weight Loss has worked for the

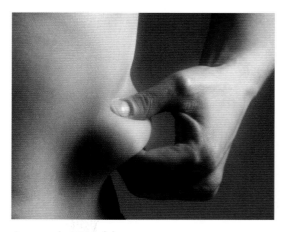

A growing problem
Obesity affects more than 300 million people world-wide – and figures show no signs of slowing down.

THE WEIGHT OF THE WORLD

Obesity is increasing on all continents and is set to become the world's biggest health problem. Here's how some countries around the world weigh in.

Country	Percentage of men who are obese	Percentage of women who are obese
Australia	18	18
Denmark	10	9
England	17	20
Finland	19	19
France	9.6	10.5
Germany	17.2	19.3
Italy	6.5	6.3
Spain	11.5	15.2
Sweden	10	11.9
USA	20	25

(Source: International Obesity Task Force. These figures are a guide only as data is constantly updated.)

thousands of patients I've treated in my New York practice. They've all lost weight, and they've maintained the weight loss. All without diets or deprivation, without starving themselves or scheduling their meals by the clock or carrying around scales to measure what they're eating – and without being angry with themselves or feeling like failures because they went out for a pizza or 'slipped up' at a party.

The first thing you need to know about your desire to lose weight is that it will happen. You are about to embark on a weight-loss programme that *will* succeed.

A WORLDWIDE PROBLEM

You are not alone in feeling unhappy about your weight. In fact, you can join a growing, worldwide crowd. From Birmingham to Brisbane, from Paris to Pretoria, in country after country and in just about every region of the planet, more than 300 million people are either overweight (defined as weighing 10 to 15 per cent above an ideal weight), or obese (20 per cent above an ideal weight), or even morbidly obese (30 per cent or more above an ideal body weight). It may be small consolation for the dismay you feel when you stand on the scales, but you're part of a global trend.

This trend is both recent and fast-moving. Around the world, the number of obese people has doubled in the last two decades. A report published by the International Obesity

You are not alone in feeling unhappy about your weight

Task Force in 2000 showed that even in China, which maintains one of the world's lowest incidences of overweight people, the growth rate in the numbers of overweight and obese people is increasing. Give the Chinese time, and weight gain will do what

FIREFIGHTING FIT

Few professions are as stressful as firefighting. Yet New York City firefighter Tom Kontizas lost 18.1kg (2st 12lb) with Picture Perfect Weight Loss. 'Without even trying', his wife Karen lost 3.6kg (8lb) just by shopping and cooking for him.

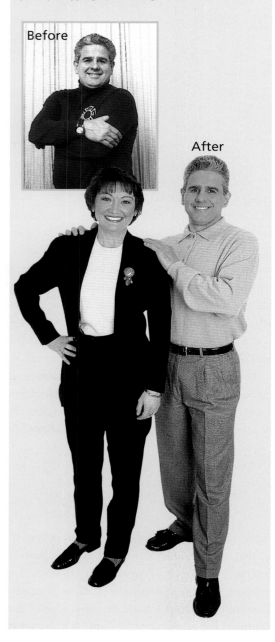

Before

After

government policy has long tried to do – decrease the billion-person population, not through population planning, but through the increased occurrence of diabetes, stroke, high blood pressure and even some forms of cancer.

TOO CLOSE FOR COMFORT

One of the countries leading the way in this unhappy, unhealthy spiral is the United Kingdom – a dubious distinction if ever there was one. Today, in 2004, it is estimated that a

> ### Dieting doesn't work – that's why you're reading this book

quarter of men and one in five women are obese, and that as many as 30,000 people in the UK die prematurely every year from obesity-related conditions.

But it's not just in the UK that the problem exists: research in Australia indicates that the country is on its way to overtaking the US as the fattest nation in the world. Obesity among Australian children has doubled in the last 10 years, hitting 20 per cent of kids.

The problem is growing rapidly. It is predicted that if the current rate of growth continues, one-third of the UK population could suffer the ill effects of excess weight within 10 to 15 years.

Chances are you know all this already. You don't really need the statistics to measure the problem. You can see it – in the office, in the supermarket, walking down the high street, in your own reflection in the mirror. And you probably don't need the dire warnings to be reminded of the ill effects of being overweight. You can feel it – in the clothes that suddenly feel tight, in your shortness of breath when you climb the stairs, in the sense of discomfort with your own body.

This discomfort is something else you share with millions. It is estimated that one in four adults in the western world are either on a diet in an attempt to lose weight or are 'watching what they eat' so they don't gain weight. We spend staggering amounts of money on trying to lose weight – on diets, on pills and supplements, by measuring out portions, counting calories, combining certain foods with certain other foods, listening to tapes, and fasting. As you know, these 'solutions' simply don't work. That's why you're reading this book.

OVERWEIGHT OR OBESE?

How did it happen? How did we get this way? How did *you* get this way?

There is one reason for becoming overweight, and there are many contributing causes. The reason is metabolic, and it is absolutely unique to the individual. Your metabolism is the particular combination of chemical processes occurring inside you. This combination, in turn, depends on the

> **Our high-stress, high-tech world affects our eating habits**

interactions occurring between genetic and environmental factors. Just what these factors are and how they interact are as distinctive to you as your fingerprint; no one else has that exact combination working in that exact way. Yet it is the sum total of all these factors and their interactions that dictates how your body handles calories, what foods taste good to you, and even how you think about food. In a sense, you've been dealt your very own metabolic hand of cards. While you may have no control over what's in the hand, you do control how you play the hand.

HOW LIFESTYLE AFFECTS US

Enter a range of additional contributing causes. These are the cultural, sociological and psychological factors that drive the lifestyle choices we all make every day – the different ways we each play our own metabolic hand of cards. These include things like the foods we eat, whether or not we exercise, and our levels of everyday stress.

Even anthropology plays a role. One important cause contributing to today's global epidemic of overweight people may simply be that, as a species, we are outstripping our own evolution. Biological anthropologists tell us that at an earlier stage of human development the ability to form fat was an advantage. When our ancestors were subject to uncontrollable cycles of feast and famine, bodies that could store fat for the lean times were 'fitter' bodies. They're the ones that survived, and as happens in evolution, the traits that kept the organism alive were the traits imprinted on the genetic code passed to descendants. The result? Humans in general evolved into organisms programmed to eat high-calorie foods they could store efficiently as fat.

Today, however, at least in the industrialised world, we aren't threatened by famine. (In those parts of the world where famine is a threat, the causes are more often than not human – typically, politics and civil unrest.) In fact, for most of us in developed countries, life is an almost endless feast. But since our bodies have evolved to deal with famine – to take in lots of calories and expend very few – our era's very abundance is a sure-fire formula for weight gain.

THE PRICE WE PAY

Other aspects of our current culture exacerbate the problem. We live in a high-stress, high-tech world. With both parents working – often long hours in high-pressure jobs – with children whose schedules would tire a marathon runner, with families in a constant state of arranging and rearranging plans for getting each family member here, there and everywhere, the idea of sitting down together for a relaxing family dinner has all but disappeared. There simply isn't time for such a meal, and even if there were, everybody is either too busy or too exhausted

> ## As we're eating more, we're exercising less

to enjoy it. It's easier, more convenient and even less costly for each family member to just pop a frozen dinner in the microwave and eat it on the run.

Meanwhile, we're increasingly equipped with mobile phones, pagers, internet access and the all-in-one remote control. Together, they let us do what we want – instantly – without even getting up out of a chair, let alone leaving home. Where our ancestors had to struggle daily to obtain sustenance, or

labour manually to earn it, we just drive to the nearest fast-food establishment – or we order a takeaway and have it delivered.

EATING OURSELVES OBESE

Fast food, in particular, is notoriously fattening. But gourmet restaurants also often rely on high-calorie ingredients and cooking methods. Their stock-in-trade, after all, is a taste experience so memorable you will find it worth the price. All too often this is achieved at the expense of your waistline. When a simple chicken breast can lift you into the realms of the sublime, it's probably because it has been topped with Gorgonzola, layered with bacon, then wrapped in puff pastry – an absolutely delicious, calorifically off-the-scale cardiac killer.

What's more – having taken a leaf out of the US book – other countries around the world are becoming increasingly accustomed to enormous portions. Huge tubs of buttered popcorn at the cinema. Litre-sized soft drinks. 'Super-sized' items that belie the phrase 'side dish'. It's as if we're proving our prosperity every time we eat.

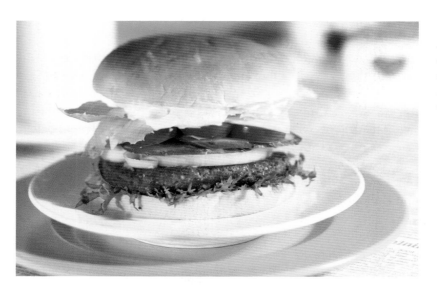

Banish the burgers
A diet of fast food combined with a lack of physical exercise is helping obesity to become the norm.

A SIDE EFFECT OF BEING OVERWEIGHT: SLEEP APNOEA

Sleep apnoea is the result of a temporary blockage of the breathing passages. Sufferers snore very loudly and actually stop breathing several times a night. Research has shown that it is most common in overweight or obese people, predominantly men, with a neck circumference of 43cm (17in) or larger. Apart from the potential consequences of the resulting daytime fatigue, there is evidence that sleep apnoea increases the risk of hypertension and heart disease. For the overweight, even a 10 per cent drop in weight can help.

TAKING THE EASY WAY OUT

Try and figure this one out: as we're eating more, we're exercising less. This, too, flies in the face of human evolution. We evolved as an active species; the human appestat, the part of the brain that regulates appetite and food

> Far too many kids prefer to be couch potatoes

intake, works best when we're active. Yet we've virtually engineered activity out of daily life – to make our lives 'easier' – everywhere and every way we can:

■ Today's workplace is increasingly automated. Machinery does most of the hauling on the factory floor, while computers in the office mean we don't even need to leave our seats to find a file or communicate with colleagues.

■ An increase in energy-saving devices in public places, such as escalators, lifts and automatic doors.

■ Cleaning chores are less labour-intensive than ever, with extendable dusters that save us from having to stretch, and powerful vacuum cleaners that mean we don't need to bend.

■ When we do go somewhere, we invariably drive, coming home to the attached garage, with doors that open automatically at the touch of a button. Even children who once walked or cycled to school or college are now driven – or some have their own cars.

■ Meanwhile, some schools have responded to budget cutbacks by reducing physical-education activities.

■ As for after school, parents in cities, in particular, find their outdoor environments too dangerous for their children to play in without supervision. Instead, they let the kids watch television or play computer games – activities that at best exercise the fingertips and at worst are accompanied by heavy snacking. Even in the suburbs, where kids have a chance to play outdoors, far too many prefer to be couch potatoes.

THE GYM MYTH

Yes, there are more gyms than ever before, more fitness videos, more newfangled pieces of exercise equipment for the home. But we tend to drive to the gym – when we actually get around to going; the videos gather dust on the shelf; and the exercise bike in the bedroom is soon obscured by the clothes we've hung on it. We actually burn 400 fewer calories per day than our great-grandparents did at the turn of the last century. On any given day, some 20 per cent of us do no physical activity that lasts longer than five consecutive minutes. That's a far cry from what we should be doing – a guideline of five sessions of 30 minutes of moderate-level exercise per week, for example.

> ## You can't fix the metabolism you were born with

All this leaves many people on a virtual treadmill that's more real than the one they hauled up to the attic years ago. On this virtual treadmill, they're running against metabolism as well as evolution, culture, sociology and a host of other contributing causes – and they're still overweight. Does this sound familiar?

WHAT DOESN'T WORK

Whatever the causes of your being overweight, in real life – *your* real life – you want to do something about it. Maybe you've tried dieting. You've measured portions and counted calories and eaten only at certain specified times of the day.

Perhaps you've tried one of the fad diets – high-protein or low-carbohydrate or no sugar or no fat. Maybe you've experimented with one or more of the new weight-loss theories that seem to crop up annually – dieting by blood type, for example, or consciously combining certain foods at certain times.

One thing these decades of changing diet fashions have demonstrated conclusively to both dieters and doctors is that the diets don't work. Sure, you lose weight at first – maybe even a lot of weight. But a diet by definition is time-limited. Unfortunately, once it's over and you return to 'real life', the weight inevitably comes back. In fact, all too often, you gain back even more than you lost in the first place. The reason is absolutely physiological: deprivation

backfires. And a diet means deprivation of all kinds as you deprive yourself of certain foods, limit your portion sizes and eat to a particular schedule rather than when you're hungry. As we'll see, forcing yourself to do what comes unnaturally eventually has the opposite effect from the one intended: not only don't you curb your appetite or eat less or lose weight, you actually become increasingly ravenous, eat more and regain what you've lost – and sometimes gain more.

DITCH THE DIET

Where diets are concerned, then, it's time to say, 'Been there, done that, got the T-shirt.' In fact, one recent study reported that dieters as a whole are fed up with all the dietary advice they're getting, especially because so much of it is conflicting advice.

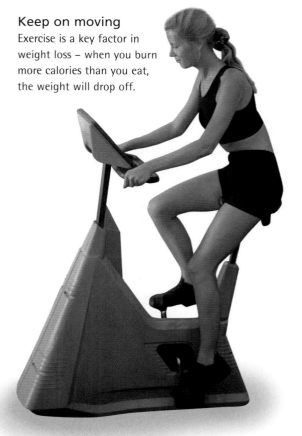

Keep on moving
Exercise is a key factor in weight loss – when you burn more calories than you eat, the weight will drop off.

They're tired of being told what to eat, when to eat it and how much of it to eat. And they're showing their anger in a backlash, eating all the foods the diet gurus and nutrition police say they shouldn't eat. It's further evidence of why diets don't work and why Picture Perfect Weight Loss *does* work: Picture Perfect Weight Loss doesn't give orders about what you should or should not eat. Instead, it provides you with a way of eating a range of foods, including the foods you love – a way of eating, *not* a diet.

But perhaps you've followed another route in order to lose weight. Maybe you bought new exercise equipment or joined the gym and began exercising to start your quest. Good for you! A consistent programme of moderate exercise is great for your fitness and sense of wellbeing. Keep it up – forever. It's very, very good for you in every way.

Or did you turn to the most recent behaviour-modification guru, the one whose calm, soothing voice on your CD player was going to 'cure' you forever of your appetite? Or maybe you swallowed the drugs or supplements that you hoped would be the ultimate 'magic bullet' leading to permanent weight loss. Neither worked. Neither *can* work.

NO SECRET TO WEIGHT LOSS

As a new wave of scientific research has confirmed time and again, there is no magic bullet with which to hit the weight-loss bull's-eye. There is no 'cure' for an individual's appetite. There is no diet format that works for everybody – or that lasts forever.

The reason that diets and pills and voices on a CD don't work is that they simply don't address the problem – that metabolic hand of cards you've been dealt. You can't fix the metabolism you were born with. When you're told what to eat, when to eat it and how much of it to eat, you're simply going against all the chemical interactions in your body. Appetite is not a disease to be 'cured'; hunger is not a whim you can repress. What we're talking about is a chemically driven message from your metabolism. If you deny it, defy it or try to silence it, chances are you simply won't be able to lose weight – or maintain the weight loss you've achieved.

WHAT DOES WORK: PICTURE PERFECT WEIGHT LOSS

There's only one way to lose weight and keep it off, and that is to change your relationship with food. What do I mean by that? I mean that you will eat when hungry, that you will eat until satisfied, that you will not exclude

> ### Appetite is not a disease to be 'cured'

from your life the foods you love. But you will eat with awareness of the consequences of what you're eating. You'll bring a big-picture approach to your eating, so that you enjoy the great variety of foods available to you while you lose weight and maintain your weight loss for life.

It's a question of choices, and the choices are all in your hands. After all, who decides what you're going to eat? Who's in charge of what you put in your mouth? Who determines how much exercise you're getting today? You do. Chances are that a lot of the choices you've been making up to now have led to the weight gain you're determined to reverse. You will reverse it – when you change the choices.

The 30-Day Plan in this book gives you the tools for change; *it will empower you.* My proven method of Food Awareness Training

(FAT) will show you the difference between food choices and make you aware of what each choice can mean. What's more, this book will show you these things in vivid demonstrations you'll see in your mind's eye every time you cook a meal or look at a menu or write your shopping list. That's Picture Perfect Weight Loss.

The programme is based on a few simple principles, and it uses a simple approach. Let's start with the three basic principles of Food Awareness Training.

■ Calorie reduction is the key to weight loss. Calories measure the energy value of food. They're one of the key determinants of whether you lose weight, stay the same or gain weight. Watching out for the fat content in foods may be an interesting exercise, but it is a useless one from the point of view of weight gain or loss. Why? Many low-fat foods are calorifically costly. *Picture Perfect Weight Loss happens when you are comfortable choosing low-calorie foods instead of high-calorie ones.* This book will show you how.

■ Choice is not deprivation. Deprivation doesn't work; in fact, it typically has the opposite effect. Starved of what you love to eat by the rules of a 'strict diet', you tend to eat voraciously once the diet is over. That's why there are no forbidden foods in Picture Perfect Weight Loss, no 'correct' portions and no specified times to eat. It's also why any reason for eating is okay. Food is not your enemy. It is a necessity that should also be a pleasure. Enjoy it!

■ You can achieve Picture Perfect Weight Loss while living your life. Maybe your life requires frequent business travel. Maybe you're home all day, taking breaks from housework by peeking into the fridge. Do you take clients to lunch? Eat breakfast on the run? Entertain a lot? Whatever your lifestyle,

tastes, needs or desires, you can still make the choices that will lead to Picture Perfect Weight Loss.

PUTTING IT INTO PRACTICE

The approach to implementing these simple principles is equally simple. In Picture Perfect Weight Loss, you *see* your food choices. What do I mean by that?

They say a picture is worth a thousand words. Turn to page 18 to see one that certainly is. On the left, there's a small amount of a high-calorie food. On the right, a huge

> **Deprivation doesn't work; it typically has the opposite effect**

amount of delicious low-calorie food. Get the picture? See, two very different sundaes – with the same number of calories. What have you learned from this demo? Four important facts:

■ Eat the food pictured on the left if you want to. No food is forbidden.

■ Eat *all* of the food pictured on the right if you want to – or if you can. Yes, you would be eating the same number of calories as the food shown on the left, but you would still be ahead. Why? Because you would be fuller – and more satisfied – than if you had eaten the high-calorie food on the left, and you'll have eaten healthier food.

■ If you eat only some of the food on the right, you're still eating more food than what's pictured on the left, but you're saving a significant number of calories.

■ Anytime you are hungry or in need of food, any food on the right is a good choice.

Above all, here is graphic evidence of the real calorific cost of the food shown on the left. The disparity in the amounts of food shown makes it clear. Obviously, the food

Are you ready to face the challenge? It's quite easy, actually. Just look at the pairs of 'food comparisons' in the pictures below and guess which food in each pair is lower in calories. The calories are based on the amount of food you see in the photographs.

Just from this short quiz, you'll get a better idea about which choices you're making the next time you see these foods. Even if you get 100 per cent correct on the quiz, the images will remind you of things that you already know about these foods. You'll discover even more, and expand your choices, as you continue reading this book.

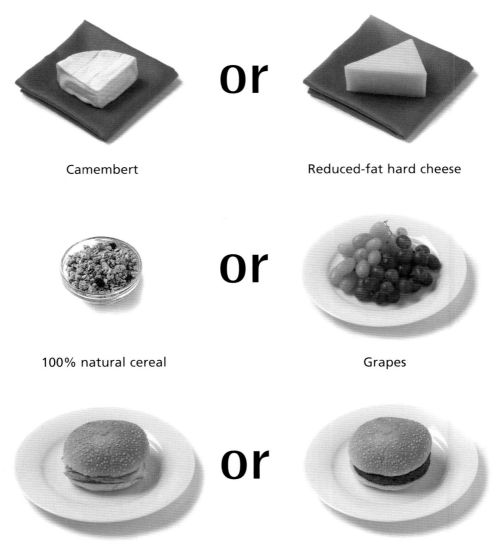

Camembert   **or**   Reduced-fat hard cheese

100% natural cereal   **or**   Grapes

Chicken burger   **or**   Veggie burger

ANSWERS TO QUIZ

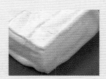 60g Camembert =
170 calories

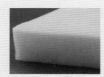 60g reduced-fat
hard cheese = 180
calories

Did you assume that the Camembert had the higher calorie count?
Many people love cheese, and we all know that it's high in fat – the kind of saturated fat we should all try to limit. The weight-conscious, however, might automatically go for the reduced-fat cheese; after all, there's something sinfully delicious about real Camembert, so we assume that it must be the high-calorie choice. But this isn't the case. Not only is it not the high-calorie choice, it's also no more packed with fat: both these cheeses contain around nine grams of largely saturated fat.

 30g 100% natural
cereal = 170
calories

 230g grapes
= 140 calories

Cereal or grapes? Read on to learn why fruit is the greater fibre provider.
Fibre is an essential component of the diet, particularly for the weight-conscious. It takes the edge off the appetite, helps fill you up for the day, and even helps to fight disease. The goal of Picture Perfect Weight Loss is to get as much fibre as possible for as few calories as possible. The best way to do that is to get your fibre from fruit and vegetables. The cereal shown here exacts a high calorie count for one gram of fibre, while this generous quantity of grapes offers three grams of fibre for fewer calories.

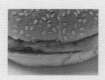 chicken burger
(120g)
= 260 calories

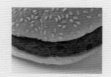 veggie burger
(120g)
= 240 calories

Think skinless chicken's healthy? Think again – soya should be your first choice.
If you thought poultry was the healthy, low-calorie alternative to beef, you should know that there's an even better alternative. Soya-based products, such as the veggie burger pictured above, are lower in calories and add the value of positive health benefits, decreasing your risk of cancer, heart disease, osteoporosis and other degenerative diseases. What's more, soya products are increasingly numerous, varied and tasty.

To convert calories to kilojoules, see page 166.

pictured on the right is not a suggested alternative to the food on the left; it's a demonstration of calorific equivalents – an exercise in awareness. The bottom line? Eat as much of the food on the right to make you feel comfortable – and you will still end up saving calories.

This book will train you in this kind of food awareness for 30 days, focusing on a different meal and/or food issue each of the four weeks. You'll see more than 50 of these demonstrations – more than 50 instances of graphic calorific evidence. By the end of the month, you'll have got the picture so perfectly you won't even need to think about your choices. *Your appetite and your taste buds will be satisfied; you won't be obsessing about food; you won't need to avoid parties or restaurants – and you will lose weight.*

And chances are you'll be saying to yourself what my patients have been saying to me in the third or fourth week of their Picture Perfect Weight Loss programmes for over 25 years: 'But Dr Shapiro, I don't even feel like I'm dieting!'

In fact, far from feeling as though they're on a diet, patients report that they do not feel deprived, are eating as much as ever (often even more than ever), are comfortable with their food choices, and are losing weight.

What has happened? In one month – just 30 days – they have simply become empowered. It's what makes Picture Perfect Weight Loss work.

THE EXERCISE FACTOR

Exercise is essential to Picture Perfect Weight Loss for reasons that are both physiological and psychological.

Physiologically, the more weight you lose the harder it can be to lose more weight. That's because the body reacts to weight loss the same way it reacts to true starvation: it actually reduces the number of calories it burns. That means that you'd have to reduce your calorie intake even further to continue to lose weight.

Burning calories through exercise helps. Exercise actually changes the way the body

> **Physical activity reduces anxiety, stress and depression**

processes food, making it easier for the body to use calories for energy rather than storing them as fat.

Perhaps just as significant is the fact that exercise helps preserve metabolically active muscle tissue. Why is this important? *(Continues on page 20.)*

HOW TO 'READ' PICTURE PERFECT DEMONSTRATIONS

Each demonstration presents at least two related food offerings. On one side is a high-calorie food or foods; on the other a lower-calorie food or foods. Typically, there will be a huge amount of the lower-calorie food. This is not meant to suggest that you should – or could! – eat that amount of low-calorie food. It's not a recommendation; it's a *demonstration*. It's meant to dramatise the point that in eating even a portion of the lower-calorie foods you will fill up, satisfy your appetite and take in fewer calories.

EVERY DAY'S A SUNDAE!

The difference between these two ice-cream sundaes can be measured in scoops – six. But of course, no one would really eat a nine-scoop sundae. Eat the same number of scoops of the reduced-fat version, get the same taste sensation, and save 120 calories.

'To dessert or not to dessert – that always seems to be the question. The choice is yours. Make it carefully, and if possible, go for the lower-calorie option.'

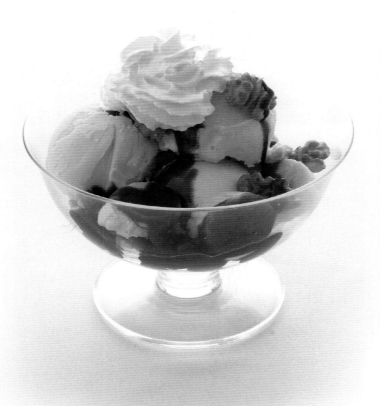

3 scoops of luxury
ice cream (180g)
300 calories **+**

walnuts (50g)
340 calories **+**

1 banana
80 calories **+**

chocolate sauce (4 tbsp)
220 calories **+**

whipped cream (20g)
60 calories
───────────────
1000 calories

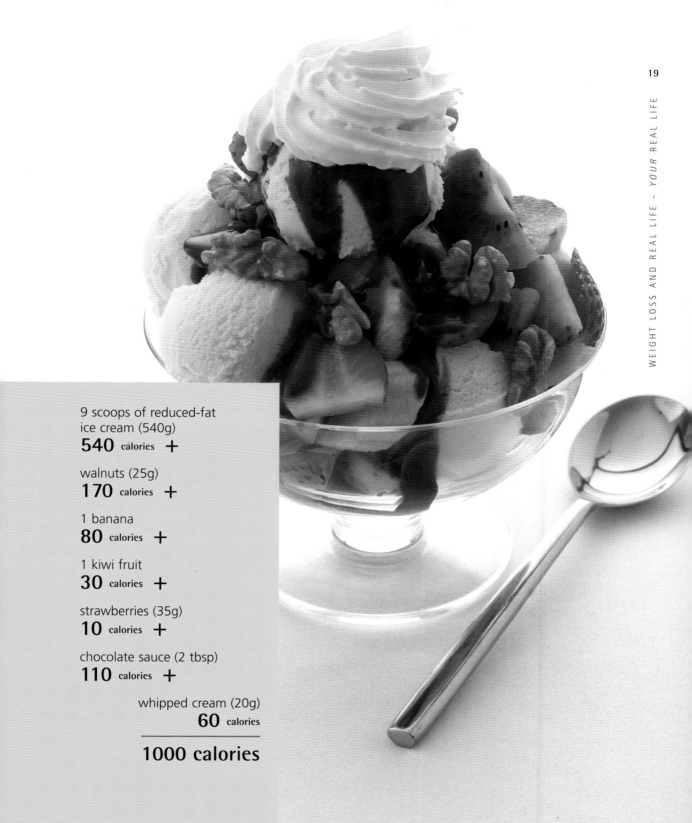

9 scoops of reduced-fat
ice cream (540g)
540 calories **+**

walnuts (25g)
170 calories **+**

1 banana
80 calories **+**

1 kiwi fruit
30 calories **+**

strawberries (35g)
10 calories **+**

chocolate sauce (2 tbsp)
110 calories **+**

whipped cream (20g)
60 calories
_____

1000 calories

Metabolically active muscle tissue uses far more calories than an equivalent weight of fat, so the more metabolically active muscle tissue you have, the higher your resting metabolic rate – that is, the number of calories your body uses when you're inactive.

Break your exercise sessions up into shorter bouts

A body that uses more calories at rest is a body that can lose weight more easily and can maintain the weight loss with only moderate calorie restriction. As if these facts weren't reason enough, exercise also acts as a temporary appetite suppressant.

Exercise has a psychological impact, too. Regular physical activity helps reduce the anxiety, stress and depression that seem to prompt overeating in many people. It 'clears the cobwebs' from the brain, lightens the mood and lifts the spirit.

ONE STEP AT A TIME

Best of all, the effect of exercise is both cumulative and pervasive. As your body becomes stronger through one form of exercise, you tend to become more physically active in other ways. You'll find yourself climbing stairs when you grow impatient with the lift, or you'll discover how much easier it has become to carry those heavy bags of groceries. It's like the old adage: the more you do, the more you *can* do. Your weight loss and your newly fit body are mutually 'encouraging', leading to a healthier, trimmer, more-active you; someone who is ready to take on more of life – and to enjoy it more.

Exercise doesn't necessarily mean jogging for an hour or getting in three sets of tennis before breakfast. Yes, high-intensity exercise certainly burns the most calories per minute, but the idea is to sustain the calorie-burning over a period of time; that's what burns the most calories over all. For that, your best bet is probably moderate- or even low-intensity exercise that you can keep doing, rather than a quick burst of all-out effort that leaves you worn out. In addition, recent research recommends breaking up exercise sessions into shorter bouts that you can repeat several times during the day. One study showed that weight loss was greater among those who ran four short stints on a treadmill than among those assigned to run one long session a day.

TAKING THE PICTURE PERFECT WEIGHT LOSS JOURNEY

Picture Perfect Weight Loss works. It worked for 26 New York City firefighters who lost between 10kg (1st 8lb) and 20.5kg (3st 3lb) over a 10-week period – and all kept on losing weight after the 10 weeks were up. You'll meet some of them in this book.

Shifting weight using Picture Perfect Weight Loss also came easily to a group of people I call the Chicago 7. In four weeks they lost between 4kg (9lb) and 9.5kg (1st 7lb) per person, with a total loss of 41kg (6st 7lb). And they're still going strong as I write this book.

The Picture Perfect Weight Loss plan has also worked for thousands of patients I've treated in my New York practice – celebrities conscious of their image, ordinary people upset about their appearance, youngsters worried about their health, and older people trying to get fit to enjoy a better and longer life.

Maybe you're allergic to certain foods – that's not a problem. Perhaps you're a senior citizen and your doctor has restricted your sodium intake or recommended that you get more calcium or focus on foods with certain

EXERCISE ARITHMETIC

Like ice cream? Then you'd better learn to like exercise, too. Here's why.

If you ate just one 60g scoop of ice cream a day for a year – and did not exercise sufficiently to burn off the extra calories in the ice cream – you would gain 4.5kg (10lb). How does it work?

Given that one 60g scoop of ice cream equals 100 calories and that 3500 excess calories are stored as 500g (1lb) of fat, calculate as follows: multiply the 100 calories per day more than your body needs by 365 days per year, then divide by the 3500 calories in a pound of fat and this gives you approximately 4.5kg (10lb).

The bottom line? If you increase your ice-cream intake, to compensate you had better increase your physical activity as well.

vitamins. You can do this with Picture Perfect Weight Loss. Maybe, because of your cultural background or religious beliefs, there are certain types of food that you grew up on and love. With Picture Perfect Weight Loss nobody will suggest that you give up those foods. On the contrary, it will lead you to a whole new range of food choices. It will expand your awareness of foods from many origins, foods of many types, foods of varying tastes.

To fully understand why so many people have lost weight by following the Picture

There's no secret involved – it's a question of empowerment

Perfect Weight Loss programme, simply study the visual demonstrations in this book. As you'll see from the photographic evidence, not one of these people has ever gone hungry. They haven't given up the foods they love. They haven't stopped cooking creatively or shopping in bulk. They eat out in restaurants with friends; they go to lunch with clients and colleagues; they enjoy power breakfasts with the boss. I'll show you the

kinds of food you can snack on, the types of food to satisfy that irresistible sweet tooth, foods to help you 'handle' holidays, and how to deal with different kinds of cuisine. You'll learn how to do all of this – with increased awareness about food and food choices.

There's no secret or magic involved. It's simply a question of empowerment – *your* empowerment. Remember the old proverb that teaches 'if you give a man a fish, you feed him a meal; if you teach a man how to fish, you feed him for life'? Picture Perfect Weight Loss teaches you to 'fish'; it's a way you can feed yourself for life. Yes, you will have to change your relationship with food; that goes without saying. But you'll incorporate this new approach comfortably, without having to change your lifestyle or your tastes, and without banging your head against a wall trying to undo the metabolic hand of cards you were dealt.

Awareness is the key – awareness of the cards in your hand and the vast universe of healthy, low-calorie food alternatives. These are all the tools you need to change your relationship with food and lose weight once and for all. After that, the choice is yours.

CHAPTER 2: PICTURE PERFECT WEIGHT LOSS THROUGHOUT LIFE

OBESITY STARTS IN CHILDHOOD

Childhood obesity is as much an epidemic as adult obesity is, and as with the grown-up version, the problem among children is widespread and growing. In the UK, from 1989 to 1998 obesity in children aged between two and four almost doubled from five per cent to nine per cent. And between 1990 and 2001, figures for kids aged between 6 and 15 trebled from 5 per cent to 16 per cent. That's a lot of weight gain, and it's a similar picture throughout the western world.

THE PRICE WE PAY

If the trends described above continue it is estimated that, at the very least, by 2020 one-fifth of boys and one-third of girls will be obese. But at what cost to themselves? As with adults, overweight children are more prone to suffer high cholesterol levels, high blood pressure and abnormal blood-sugar counts. And that's not all. They are at serious risk of cardiovascular disease, diabetes and other chronic ailments.

Chairman of the International Obesity Task Force Professor Philip James thinks we're heading for disaster unless we quickly change the way we approach how our children eat and exercise: 'The first step must be to start protecting the health and well-being of our young children, who are being damaged because we are not yet willing to provide them with a safe environment where they can experience and learn the value of good food and play,' says Professor James.

One of the starkest facts about overweight children is that they tend to grow into overweight adults. In the UK, overweight young people have a 50 per cent chance of being overweight adults, and children of overweight parents have twice the risk of being overweight compared to those with healthy weight parents.

While scientists are pretty certain of the main reasons why children today are overweight – a lack of physical activity, thanks to television and computer games, combined

> **Overweight children tend to grow into overweight adults**

with too much of too many high-calorie foods – they don't really know why being overweight in the growing years tends to lead to being overweight as adults. Part of the reason may be as much psychological as physiological. Perhaps overweight children simply accept their weight as a normal condition – especially if excess weight is something they see in a beloved parent or role model. Or maybe overweight kids simply get into the 'habit' of being overweight.

An unhealthy cycle develops. Because the child is overweight, it's harder for him or her to exercise or to enjoy sports. So the child stays on the sidelines while the other kids are burning up calories. That adds even more weight – and makes it that much harder to exercise. And so it goes, on and on.

THE PAIN OF BEING AN OVERWEIGHT CHILD

Seriously overweight or obese children can pay a high price for their condition. The psychological and emotional toll as well as the physical cost can be enormous – and can have lifelong consequences.

There's no point in tiptoeing around the issue; overweight children know they are overweight. They get the message every day, perhaps from their parents at home or other children in the playground, and at this important stage of their development the message can produce a long-lasting sense of inferiority and insecurity.

Beyond school and home, of course, the media bombard all of us with images of how we're supposed to look. Young children are more likely than adults to embrace these images as a standard to admire and emulate, and for overweight children it's abundantly clear they don't look the way they're 'supposed to'. One disturbing result of this is

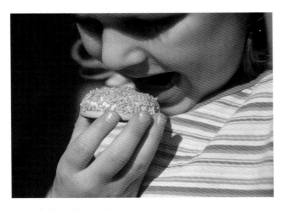

Food for thought
Childhood obesity has never been so prevalent – it's time to change our approach to food and exercise.

that younger and younger children are worried about their own body image, particularly their weight, and, tragically, more and more young children are falling victim to eating disorders.

No wonder anorexia and bulimia, the serious, occasionally fatal, diseases usually associated with adolescence, are now seen in children – especially girls – sometimes as

> **A dislike of their bodies can set kids on a dangerous path**

young as eight years old. But even for youngsters who aren't affected by these dreadfully harmful disorders, a dislike of their own bodies can set children on other dangerous paths – fasting, for example, or the kind of dieting that deprives children of the necessary foods and nourishment they need for growth and maturation as well as for all-around good health.

UNDERSTANDING THE ISSUE

What should you do if your child is overweight? That's the heart of the issue – and the issue is multifaceted and complex.

First of all, it's important to note that not every overweight child is an unhealthy child – or destined to become an overweight, unhealthy adult. Weight gain is very much a part of growing up, and a plentiful variety of foods is essential to the process of building strong bones and muscles.

Especially in the period just before puberty, and especially in girls, weight gain – even considerable weight gain – is absolutely normal and may be desirable. This is just one reason why all that body-image scrutiny on the part of young girls is so troubling. If a pre-pubescent girl diets her way through this important growth phase, the results can be disastrous. Some young girls have gone so far as to stave off the onset of their menstrual cycles by simply not eating, or by not eating

> ## Parents' attitudes towards food influence their children

enough healthy foods. Both physiologically and psychologically, this resistance to eating is worrying and needs to be overcome.

FEAR OF FOOD

Parents' attitudes towards food also influence their children's behaviour. Parents are role models; their food habits tend to become their kids' food habits, and how they approach eating can influence their children for life. So many of the patients who come to my office in New York have vivid memories of their mothers restricting certain foods because they were fattening or pushing certain other foods because they were considered healthy. Food thus instantly became a kind of dividing line, a standard of behaviour. In many ways, the use

of food became frightening. Patients tell of asking for an after-school snack and being told they could have 'a' snack but not the snack they wanted; instead, many bought the forbidden food secretly with pocket money from the local shops.

TO DIET OR NOT TO DIET?

What should the parents of an overweight child do? How should you handle the food situation at home? Should you seek 'treatment' for your child? Is there a single solution that works? Should you put your child on a diet or not?

Doctors, paediatricians, psychologists and nutritionists approach this issue from varying perspectives, but all are pretty much agreed that while action can be advisable, putting kids on a diet tends to do more harm than good. For one thing, where young children are concerned, restricting foods only makes those foods more attractive, while forcing a particular food on a child typically backfires, actually creating an aversion to that food. Even more importantly, a diet is a treatment programme that measures success or failure.

BODY MASS INDEXING FOR CHILDREN

A healthy weight has a very positive effect on our well-being. The healthy-weight range is based on a measurement known as the Body Mass Index (BMI). This is calculated by dividing body weight in kilograms by the square of height in metres. Higher BMIs usually point to an increase in body fat and excess weight. A BMI of 20–24.9 represents a healthy weight; 25–29.9 is overweight; and a BMI of 30 or higher is recognised as being obese.

Now BMI has been incorporated into growth charts for children as young as two, providing doctors with an important tool for identifying those with the potential to become overweight or obese. BMI gives paediatricians and doctors treating patients up to the age of 20 the chance to intervene when necessary to prevent significant medical problems in adulthood and deal with more immediate self-esteem problems, such as eating disorders.

LEARNING DISABILITY

Do you ever overeat? Many of us do when we dine out, celebrate a birthday or sit down to Christmas dinner. But why? Maybe we've *learned* to. A group of three-year-olds ate only as much pasta as they needed until they were satiated, no matter how much was put on their plates. A group of five-year-olds ate more when given larger portions. The conclusion? According to nutrition researcher Barbara Rolls, PhD, of Pennsylvania State University, learned behaviour overtakes instinct between the ages of three and five. While the body instinctively would stop eating when satisfied, we learn to choose the biggest slice of cake.

Putting your child on a diet, therefore, adds the pressure of 'performance' to all the other pressures he or she is feeling. And since diets almost always end in failure, forcing a kid to

> ### Forcing kids to go on a diet will only make them miserable

go on one holds the danger of simply adding to his or her misery – the last thing you want for your child.

As with adults, there's another way to help your overweight child. Simply put: apply the principles of Picture Perfect Weight Loss.

PICTURE PERFECT WEIGHT LOSS FOR CHILDREN

Start by determining whether your child is experiencing normal growth or if his or her weight is actually a health risk. Visit your doctor, who may refer you to a paediatrician. Putting on weight before puberty is completely normal; this may just be a little puppy fat – extra weight that will drop off as soon as your child discovers football or sprouts another few centimetres.

But if there is a problem, it's extremely important to understand it – and to present it to your child – as a health issue, an issue of nutrition. For one thing, in doing so, you are starting from a position of love. You're saying something nurturing to your child – 'This is good for you' – instead of implying that the child weighs too much. The former can be encouraging; the latter only damages your child's self-image and sense of self-worth. In fact, throughout your child's Picture Perfect Weight Loss programme, it is essential that he or she receive consistent and total acceptance, approval and encouragement.

Second, by understanding this as a *health issue*, not a treatment programme, you take

GET THEM MOVING

Check out the following practical suggestions to get children away from the computer or television – and, in the process, get them excited about doing physical activities.

- ◆ Get off the internet, go to a real library.
- ◆ Encourage face-to-face conversations, not just the use of email.
- ◆ Sign your child up for after-school sports, music or arts clubs, or community activities.
- ◆ Use weekends constructively and organise outdoor family activities.

away the pressure. With Picture Perfect Weight Loss, you're not asking the child to lose weight or even to reduce calories. That's just the sort of thing that lends itself to measurement – and to failure. Instead, you're encouraging your child to make changes. It's a life lesson, not a corrective action.

Finally, what's particularly important about Picture Perfect Weight Loss for children is the same thing that sets it apart for adults: Picture Perfect Weight Loss is an approach that *empowers the child* to make choices that will be comfortable. Yes, it accomplishes the calorie reduction the child needs to lose weight, but it does so without the deprivation that is always a problem for kids – and that invariably backfires.

Change *is* possible – and it works. The younger people are when they change their relationship with food, the better off they will be. Where kids are concerned, it's up to the parents to get the change underway.

SOCIAL FORCES ENCOURAGE CHILDHOOD WEIGHT GAIN

Food manufacturers spend hundreds of millions of pounds a year targeting young children in their advertising and marketing of fast-food meals, sugar-rich biscuits, cakes and sweets, and high-calorie/low-nutrition drinks and snacks. Fast-food chains are quick to buy advertising slots during children's programming and focus on selling them the latest food fad, often endorsed by a cuddly cartoon character. This combined force of television and advertising works.

> ## Picture Perfect is a life lesson, not a corrective action

Children have responded: they love 'junk foods', and for today's families where both parents work, a fast-food family dinner may be all they have time for. But what effect are these images of burgers, biscuits, crisps and sweets having on our children? Could they contribute to the onset of obesity in later life?

To make matters worse, kids are less active than ever before. Many schools have responded to budget cutbacks by reducing or even eliminating physical education – or by closing gym facilities. With two parents

---

THE TELEVISION TRAP

Television is a major culprit in both encouraging kids to eat junk food and preventing them from exercising. Studies show that kids watch a huge amount of television, and British children are some of the worst offenders. Kids in the UK aged six to 16 spend around three hours a day in front of the television compared to two hours elsewhere in Europe.

Meanwhile, in Australia, a new study into children's television viewing habits reveals fast food companies have overtaken toy manufacturers in deliberately targeting young people with advertising on television. With obesity currently affecting one in five Australian teenagers, the outlook is bleak unless changes are made.

As if to compound these findings, in a recent US study researchers have found a correlation between the number of hours of television watched and a child's body mass index and body fatness. (Body Mass Index, or BMI, is a measure that takes into account a person's weight and height to measure total body fat; it's a good way to determine when extra weight translates into health risks. *See page 24*.) Children in the higher viewing brackets – watching four hours or more per day – had a greater BMI than those who watched less than two hours.

A YOUNG BOY'S PAIN - AND PROGRESS

They came to see me as a family – mother, father and 10-year-old son, Andrew. All three needed and wanted to lose weight, but the catalyst that actually propelled them into my office was Andrew. Even for a boy who excelled in his studies, loved sports and was popular with his friends, weight had become an issue.

The issue? 'Just looking at yourself in the mirror,' Andrew told me, 'and being able to keep up with kids when you're running.' For an avid cricket fan who doubles as a bowler and batsman, athletic ability is certainly an essential quality. As for looking at himself in the mirror and not liking what he saw, it turns out that Andrew had help in that: one day, a classmate insulted him by calling him a name. Even for a popular kid with high self-esteem, the impact was devastating.

Andrew's parents chose to support his wish to lose weight by going on the Picture Perfect Weight Loss programme with him. For all three, there has been substantial progress. Andrew has made very real changes in his eating habits – and he is proud of himself for having done so. These days his lunch box usually contains tuna with lettuce and tomato in a roll, a piece of fruit for dessert and a lollipop for an extra snack. When he goes to McDonald's – his favourite restaurant, as it is for most children his age – Andrew finds he is just as happy tucking into a tossed salad with light dressing and grilled chicken as he used to be indulging in a Big Mac.

This young man is changing his relationship with food, doing things differently for himself, losing weight and feeling very good about himself. And that's not all: another positive result of following the Picture Perfect Weight Loss programme is that Andrew is also getting healthier, and he thinks that's important, too.

working, outdoor play is discouraged because neither parent is available to supervise the children's safety. And many kids simply resist sports or playing outdoors in favour of games consoles and surfing the internet.

Many schools have reduced or eliminated physical education

Put all these social and cultural changes together, and it's no wonder childhood obesity has reached epidemic proportions. Is there a solution to this problem? Of course there is. First, children need to get up and get moving. Parents can play a vital part in encouraging this: get outside with your kids and get fit! Why not walk down to the local park and have a game of football, or do some light jogging together, or go swimming as a family once a week? Fly a kite. Even walking the dog needn't be a chore if you find new areas to roam and start exploring.

Children also need to turn to alternative, low-calorie food choices. Want an idea? Turn the page. You'll also find many more food choices suitable for kids dotted throughout the rest of the book. And try to encourage your children to try new foods; that way they'll receive more of the benefits on offer.

LUNCH BOX FUN?

Just how much fun is a small lunch that costs your child 550 calories — much of it from fat and refined carbohydrates? The lunch on the right offers considerably more food and is far healthier, providing your child with a great source of protein from the tuna. Just as importantly, this more nutritionally rewarding lunch does not set your child apart as 'different' or 'on a diet'. Maybe it's time to redefine 'fun'.

'Don't talk about foods as being "good" or "bad" – rather, talk about foods that nourish us.'

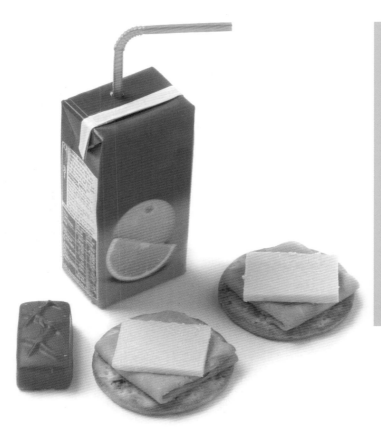

hard cheese (50g)
200 calories **+**

ham (30g)
35 calories **+**

crackers
120 calories **+**

orange juice (200ml)
95 calories **+**

chocolate bar (20g)
100 calories
———————————
550 calories

VS

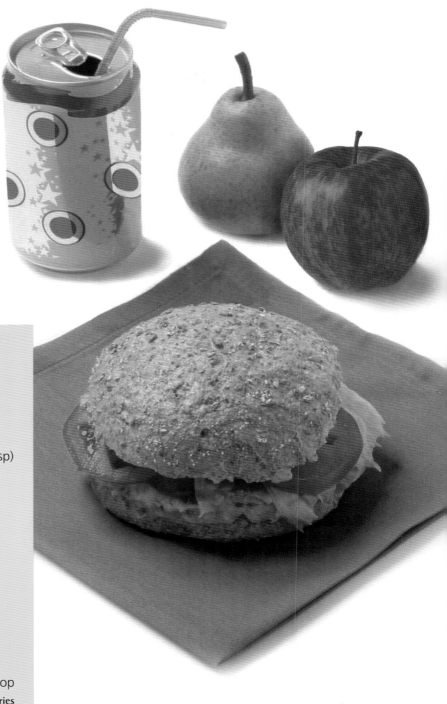

wholemeal roll (50g)
125 calories **+**

tuna (75g)
75 calories **+**

low-fat creamy dressing (1 tbsp)
30 calories **+**

lettuce and tomato garnish
10 calories **+**

diet cola (330ml)
0 calories **+**

pear
50 calories **+**

apple
50 calories **+**

lollipop
50 calories

_____

390 calories

THE DANGEROUS TEENS

Now I want to speak directly to all the teenagers out there. I know that you're concerned about your appearance – who isn't? – and that this concern is often related to your weight. I also know that social life has become all-important, and that a great deal of

> ### A great deal of teenage social life revolves around food

teenage social life revolves around food. The question is, how can you reconcile the concern about your weight with all that eating? And, just as important, how can you do it without drawing attention to yourself?

Picture Perfect Weight Loss provides the answers to these questions and many more using the food-comparison demonstration in this chapter and the others featured throughout this book. These low-calorie choices let you satisfy your hunger (which is pretty big at this point in life), fit in with the crowd (also an important goal), and lose weight or stay slim at the same time.

After you've looked at enough of the food demos, you'll get the picture. You'll be able to adjust your relationship with food in such a way that you can feel comfortable in just about any situation involving food – while still doing your best for your appearance and, more importantly, for your health.

DO YOU WANT TO BE THIN?

Of course you want to be thin. *Everybody* wants to be thin. Being overweight just isn't cool. Neither is drawing attention to your weight by dieting when everyone else is eating everything they want *when* they want.

If you're an adolescent girl, 'thin is in' is a message that is drummed into your head loudly and constantly almost around the

Teenagers today
Body image is often high on the list of teenagers' concerns, and this can lead to weight issues.

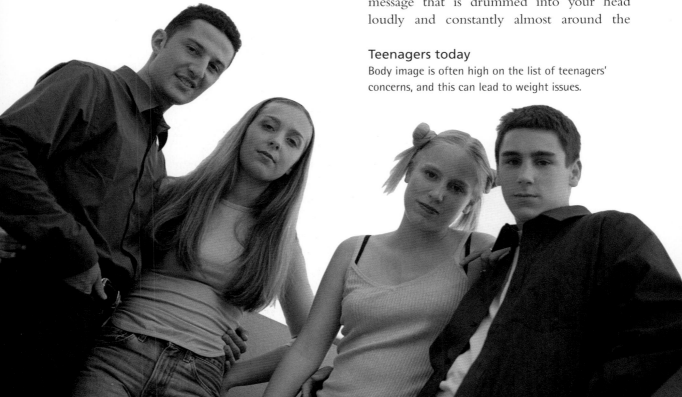

clock. A study of one teen magazine over two decades found that every single article expressed the idea that losing weight would make you prettier – every single article, for 20 years. The fact that weight loss might make you fit and healthy was barely mentioned.

GETTING THE PICTURE

The picture that TV commercials are painting – the picture just about everything in our culture is painting – is one in which thinness equates to success and power and everything else admirable and desirable. It's a particular kind of thinness, too. I don't know if you ever read the high-fashion, high-design magazines, but the ads in those magazines feature emaciated-looking women and men. Their

> **TV commercials tell us that thinness equates to success**

bones protrude. Their skin seems tissue-thin. Of course, the stylists who create these ads intensify the look with grey, flat tones that accentuate attenuated bodies. But the point they're trying to make is that this is the look you're supposed to think is the height of fashion, the appearance to strive for.

Well here's a statistic for you: the supermodels who may be your ideal of how a woman should look are thinner than 98 per cent of the female population of the western world. In fact, where the average fashion model is 1.8m (5ft 11in) tall and weighs 53.1kg (8st 4lb), the average woman is 1.62m (5ft 4in) tall and weighs about 63.5kg (10st). That's quite a discrepancy. One look is fake and contrived, the other real. But you see so much of the artificial look that you may have trouble seeing the difference – or you just may not care. You've got the message: thin is where it's at.

ACTING ON THE MESSAGE

Maybe you are overweight. If so, of course you want to be thinner. So you've decided to go on a diet. But which one? Believe me, it doesn't matter. Whichever diet you choose, one thing is certain: it won't work.

Oh, you may indeed lose weight – at first. Any rigid eating plan will eventually reduce your total intake of calories, and calories are the main determining factor in weight loss. One reason your calorie intake goes down is the monotony of the diet. But weight lost through dieting invariably comes right back. How do I know? I've seen it in literally thousands of patients; they come to me because they're tired of the up-and-down cycle – dieting to lose weight, putting it back on, dieting again, putting it back on again. They want to get off the roller coaster and find a new way of eating that will get them thin and keep them thin.

It is estimated that 95 per cent of dieters regain their lost weight and more within five years of dieting. Not only that, studies also show that the next time you try to diet, it becomes harder to lose weight . . . and harder still every successive time you try to diet. The reason? Mother Nature tenaciously guards the fat stored within you as a protection against starvation. When you go on a diet and wilfully restrict your food intake, she reacts by slowing down your metabolism. Not only won't you keep off the weight you lose on the diet, you'll actually put on more.

One result of restrictive dieting can be nutritional deficiencies that are downright bad for your health and that can have long-lasting effects. Another result is that you can actually knock your body chemistry out of sync and mess up the mind-body link – no longer even recognising your own hunger signs. Obviously, this can also have a long-lasting impact.

At this point, you're probably wishing I would mind my own business. But that's exactly what I *am* doing. I'm a doctor, after all. Your health, particularly if you want to lose weight, is the business I'm in. And I know what you're going to say next, too – that 'everybody diets'. I will agree that dieting has become a recognised pastime in the western world, but that doesn't mean it's not harmful. And the negative health effects are far more enduring than the ephemeral shedding of weight.

HOW TO LOSE WEIGHT – FOR REAL

You want to lose weight? There's a wrong way to do it and a right way to do it. Inappropriate eating is the wrong way and can lead to results that may haunt you for the rest of your life. Why? There are two reasons: one, with inappropriate eating, you fail to take in the proper amounts of nutrients you need; two, inappropriate eating is restrictive eating – that is, you deprive yourself of

There's a wrong way and a right way to lose weight

certain foods and limit your intake of others. This kind of restrictive eating can actually condemn you to weight gain.

Why is getting the right amount of nutrients so essential? I'm sure you know the answer to this already: nutrients are what keep the body working. Protein is the essential body-building nutrient, used to manufacture and repair all the body's cells. Carbohydrates are the primary source of energy. Fats are the fuel for such chemical activities as growth, metabolism and the manufacture of sex

MEETING THE NEEDS FOR CALCIUM AND IRON

Any parent of a teenager is familiar with the growth spurt. Occurring somewhere between the ages of 12 and 18, often in increments, almost always noisily, the adolescent growth spurt is a true physiological phenomenon. In fact, it is estimated that 45 per cent of an individual's skeletal growth occurs at this time. To fuel the growth of both bone and muscle, the body needs twice the amount of calcium and iron it normally requires.

One consequence of this growth spurt is that teens require adequate amounts of both calcium and iron in their diets. The need for calcium is obvious: it's the essential ingredient of all that skeletal growth. As for the iron, boys need it for the build-up of muscle mass, a

process that requires a high volume of blood. Girls need iron, too; their menstrual periods begin, and they need to replenish the iron lost in each monthly flow.

Say 'iron' in connection with food, and most people think of a juicy steak or hamburger. Say 'calcium', and just about everybody thinks of milk or cheese. But meat and dairy products are not the best or healthiest ways to consume iron and calcium. Both can start the ball rolling for a range of conditions later in life, and both can be high-calorie. Instead, teenagers should aim to get their calcium and iron from soya products, pulses and green vegetables.

hormones. Minerals build bones and teeth. Vitamins fight disease. We need them all.

For teenagers, these nutrients are particularly important. Without adequate amounts of all these nutrients, you're short-changing your body at what is a critical stage in your physical, sexual and mental growth. This is a time of major bone and muscle growth, and it's the time when the sexual organs are developing to maturity. Inadequate nutrition can affect all of these things. In fact, inadequate amounts of nutrients can adversely impact on every body process, your overall physical performance, even your mental acumen.

> ## Eliminating any one nutrient is both foolish and scary

How? You lose muscle strength, dilute your stamina and lower your body's use of oxygen. This in turn can result in dehydration and electrolyte imbalances, and it can even make you lose co-ordination.

Mentally, the mind's reaction times slow. It becomes harder to concentrate. And while some people eat to excess because they're depressed or anxious, dieting inappropriately can cause similar feelings.

KEEP YOUR BALANCE

In many cases, the adverse impact of inappropriate eating can be permanent. With girls in particular, if the percentage of your body fat goes below a certain critical level, this can interfere with the balance of female hormones. This, in turn, can affect or even eliminate menstruation and may affect your ability to have children later on.

Now you know why nutritionists always advise eating a balanced diet. Obviously,

limiting or eliminating any one nutrient – as the high-protein, low-carb diets suggest – is both foolish and scary. A balanced diet is a varied diet, one that gives you all the nutrients your body needs and gives them to you in the amounts you need – as a teenager – for growth and maturation.

The other wrong way to lose weight through inappropriate eating is by restricting certain kinds of food or limiting amounts. It can be dangerous, and here's how it can hurt: studies show that if you don't respond to your own personal food needs – eating food you like, when you want it, in the amount that satisfies you – you can actually do damage to your body's weight-regulating mechanism. Your metabolism slows, and your body responds as if fighting starvation, closing down functions in order to save energy. When this 'famine response' kicks in, it affects your psyche and causes a pattern of disordered eating, an obsession with food and, almost invariably, weight gain.

In fact, when you feel deprived of food, that's a message from your metabolism. The

BODY IMAGE, BODY DAMAGE

A survey of 2000 girls for *Bliss* magazine found six out of 10 would be happier if they lost weight. The survey revealed that while 19 per cent of those questioned were overweight, 67 per cent thought they needed to lose weight. Of those who wanted to lose weight, some 46 per cent wanted to lose more than 6.4kg (1st). Editor Helen Johnson says it is 'tragic' that so many girls want to be thin. 'Female body image obsession has grown year on year since the 60s and it has now reached epidemic proportions, filtering down to young girls,' she explains. 'Now many girls of 13 and 14 are dieting constantly at an age when their bodies are still developing.'

message is, I'm now going to kick you up the backside and actually make you *gain* weight. Why gain weight? Because you're defying your body's natural hunger, throwing your

If you don't respond to your food needs you can do damage

internal weight-regulating mechanism out of kilter, and in a sense messing with your body's intrinsic balance. Your body will fight back; it sets in motion the disordered thinking and eating that lead to weight gain.

EAT FOOD, LOSE WEIGHT

The only way to lose weight and keep it off is to take in fewer calories than you burn up. How can you do this while ensuring you get all the nutrients you need and without depriving yourself? When your body tells you to eat, eat a healthy, low-calorie food.

'Okay,' I hear you saying, 'but what if my brain instructs me to eat a 500ml tub of luxury chocolate ice cream?' What my Picture

Perfect Weight Loss programme is all about is showing you that there are alternatives to a 500ml tub of luxury chocolate ice cream. There are lower-calorie choices that you will find appetising, and they're pictured throughout this book. For the same number of calories in that 500ml tub of luxury chocolate ice cream, for example, you could eat 45 chocolate milk ice lollies – same chocolate taste, similar creaminess. Or you could have 1 litre of sorbet.

Of course, you probably can't eat 45 chocolate milk ice lollies. Chances are you would eat only one or two – maybe even three. And you would probably want only a few scoops of sorbet. Therefore, by opting for the lower-calorie choice, you are automatically taking in fewer calories. The result? You can get and stay thin by eating food you enjoy. *Picture it: you can lose weight by eating food you like when you're hungry and until you're satisfied. That is the right way to lose weight, and it is at the heart of Picture Perfect Weight Loss.*

It's simple. Check out the food comparison demonstration on the opposite page.

UNSAFE SPEED

A popular drug of choice among teenagers because of its appetite-suppressing properties, amphetamines – also called speed, whiz, uppers, amph, billy, sulphate, grudge, blues, bennies, crazy horse and jollies – stimulate the central nervous system.

Amphetamines were originally used in the 1930s as a treatment for colds, flu and hay fever, but their use has changed today. Under medical supervision, these drugs have been used to treat depression, obesity and other

conditions; in non-medical or 'recreational' use, they keep people awake and may briefly improve athletic performance. Eventually, users of these drugs are likely to become compulsive, suspicious and disorganised. Over the long term, they may develop serious mental and physical illnesses.

The abuse of amphetamines in order to lose weight is entirely discredited. It can lead to malnutrition and dangerous weight loss, and withdrawal can be difficult. Plus it's illegal.

PACK A SNACK WITH FRUIT

When teenagers are hungry for something to nibble on, the likelihood is they'll reach for snack foods. And why not? They require no cooking, you only have to open the packet – and they're delicious! But some choices can carry a high cost in calories. Take these peanuts, for instance. You'll have much more to munch on – and for longer – by choosing the popcorn and grapes, and you'll take in some fruit as well.

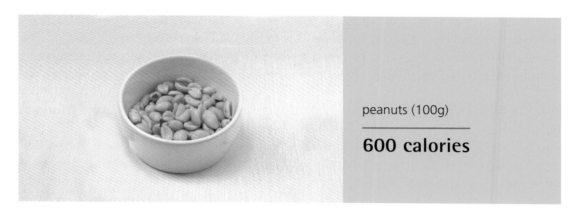

peanuts (100g)
_____

600 calories

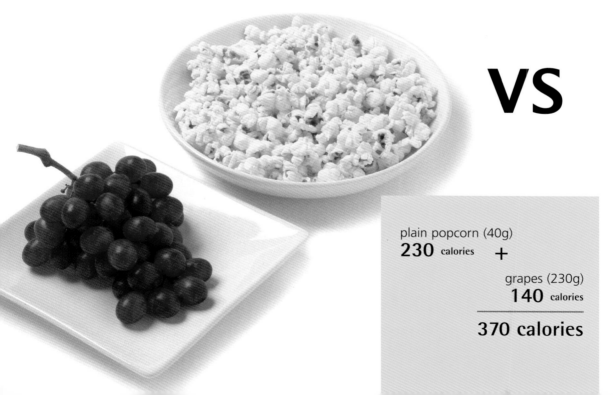

VS

plain popcorn (40g)
230 calories **+**

grapes (230g)
140 calories
_____

370 calories

MOVING INTO THE MIDDLE YEARS AND BEYOND

Welcome to the middle years. If you're somewhere between the ages of 30 and 55, chances are that you woke one morning to find that you had put on a little weight. Possibly even a lot of weight.

I'll bet it sneaked up on you. One day, you just happened to notice that your clothes felt snug, or that the person looking back at you from the mirror was unrecognisable, or that you weren't moving with the ease you once took pride in. You found you suddenly felt uncomfortable in your own body. Once upon a time, you could eat any food in any amount and never put on weight. Not any more.

YOUR SLOWING METABOLISM

While every individual is different, the middle years in general are a time of small, incremental physiological changes that all too often lead to weight gain. Simply put, your metabolism slows, and it begins to show in your waistline. Your body just isn't burning calories the way it used to. It's easier to put weight on, harder to take weight off. It's not fair, but it's also not your fault.

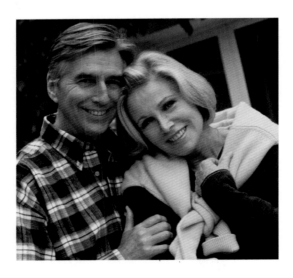

Put some of the blame on lifestyle. If you have a job or career, these are your peak earning years. This usually means stress, and

> ## The middle years all too often lead to weight gain

stress in turn is typically a good excuse for bad eating habits. Maybe you're on the go, travelling frequently for business, eating as and when you can, with neither the time to exercise nor access to exercise facilities. Maybe you wolf down lunch at your desk while answering phones that never stop ringing, trying to keep people happy and keep up with your workload – all of which leaves you feeling simultaneously stuffed and dissatisfied, not to mention suffering from a bad case of heartburn. Or perhaps you dine lavishly with clients, courtesy of a generous expense account, mixing rich food with the need to strike a business deal and close it.

Relationships can become stressed, too, especially because the constant logistical hassles and the separate work lives of husband and wife can leave little time for intimacy or romance. This is a vulnerable time of life. All too often, it's a time when people form bad eating habits – eating for comfort, eating through stress, eating what's fast and easy.

THE THREAT OF DISEASE

You've been eating unhealthily for a while, but you've never really paid it much attention. Then one day you hear a siren or see an ambulance zoom by and you're surprised to realise it's for the guy who lives down your

The middle years of your life
Now isn't the time to neglect your diet or to stop exercising – it's time to take care of yourself.

street or the woman in the flat upstairs – someone who is the same age as you. You begin to think about the possibility that you, too, could become ill. Suddenly, diseases like hypertension and heart disease, diabetes, osteoporosis and cancer – all these debilitating, degenerative ailments – don't seem so far-fetched.

How can you decrease your own risk of disease? The studies you read about in the newspapers tell you that what you eat today can directly affect your level of risk of these diseases and ailments. They make it clear that a diet that's based on a wide range of fruit and vegetables and that gets its protein from pulses, seafood and soya rather than from meats and dairy is the best way to lower the risk of degenerative disease. Such a diet is at the heart of Picture Perfect Weight Loss.

Of course, risk is individual. So is the weight issue, and it is different at different stages of the middle years and for populations of different countries. Still, for many people at the midpoint of life, weight gain can cause serious concern. Picture Perfect Weight Loss offers a healthy, sensible, satisfying solution whatever the circumstances.

LOSE WEIGHT – AND KEEP IT OFF – IN THE MIDDLE YEARS

However the middle years affect you – whatever your situation, whatever the crisis of the moment – eating in response to these events can cause weight gain at a time of life when it is harder than ever to shed extra bulk. If there's one life lesson we should all have learned by middle age, it's that actions have consequences. In the middle years, eating without awareness and failing to exercise adequately bring consequences that are difficult to undo. The weight doesn't shift as easily as it used to.

There is often a psychological trigger for this kind of mindless eating, yet the consequences of the eating only exacerbate the depression. There are often work-related reasons for eating, but the business can be accomplished just as effectively over a healthy, low-calorie meal. As for the insistence that there is 'no time for exercise', there's a simple answer to that: find time. Make the time. Make exercise an integral part of your life. In Chapter 3 of

The weight doesn't shift as easily as it used to

this book, I'll lay out a programme of exercise, but no programme is sufficient in a culture in which gadgets make it possible to do just about anything without getting up out of your chair. Instead, we must learn to incorporate exercise into our lives – by taking the stairs instead of the lift, by cycling rather than driving to work, by taking a brisk walk during your lunch hour, or by mowing the lawn or raking leaves. Half an hour of moderate activity a day is recommended, but if you can't do a solid half hour, how about a 10-minute walk back to the office from lunch, a walk up at least a couple of flights of the office stairs, and another brisk 10-minute walk in the evening?

FIBRE MAY FIGHT DIABETES

There's new evidence that consuming 50 grams of fibre per day – that's nearly three times the UK government's recommended daily intake of 18 grams – can lower blood sugar levels in people with Type 2, or adult-onset, diabetes. Lowering your blood sugar levels can delay or prevent such complications as blindness, lower-leg amputations and heart disease.

GIVE CALORIES THE BURN

Picture Perfect Weight Loss works even more powerfully when exercise is an integral part of your life. Of course, that's primarily because exercise burns calories. But there's more to it than that; the weight lost through exercise is weight that tends to stay lost as long as the exercise is continued. So think of exercise as an absolutely essential component not just of your Picture Perfect Weight Loss programme but of your life.

The middle years are crucial. They weigh on the mind – and can weigh on the body. But if you can use these crucial years to make both food awareness and the exercise components of Picture Perfect Weight Loss daily habits, you'll maintain weight loss – and fitness – forever. And remember: this is *only* the middle period of your life. The good habits you get into now can set you up for a whole new lease of life as you grow older.

NUTRIENTS AND NO-NO'S FOR OLDER PEOPLE

While all nutrients are essential at every stage of life for everyone, for older people approaching retirement age, the usual recommendations to eat plenty of fruit and vegetables and to go easy on meat and dairy are especially pertinent.

Both older men and women should think twice before downing a glass of milk or indulging a passion for cheese or other dairy products. Recent studies have shown that two substances that occur together in many dairy

> ## Good habits can set you up for a whole new lease of life

products – oestrogen and IGF-1, an insulin-like growth factor – encourage the growth of cancer cells, particularly breast and prostate cancer. Researchers found, for example, that men with higher levels of IGF-1 were more likely to develop prostate cancers than men with low levels of IGF-1.

So how can you take in the calcium you need without eating dairy products? The answer is simple: soya foods, leafy green vegetables, nuts, pulses and fortified cereals give you all the calcium you need more effectively and more healthily than dairy foods – and at a far lower cost in calories.

THE 'SPARE TYRE' IN WOMEN

Weight gain around the middle of the body is an issue that concerns many women in mid-life, and the 'spare tyre' that is gained can be dangerous. Why? Doctors think that the particular kind of fat that accumulates at the waistline contributes to high blood pressure and higher blood levels of cholesterol.

What causes the spare tyre? One key factor is the decline in levels of growth hormone and oestrogen during menopause; a second factor is a possible rise in levels of the stress hormone cortisol, which both increases appetite and sends the extra calories directly to the belly – just where it isn't wanted. Confirming this theory, Swedish researchers have found that stressed-out monkeys had high cortisol levels, over-ate and developed abdominal obesity.

MENOPAUSE AND WEIGHT GAIN

Many women start to put on weight during the menopause, which is another reason why diet and exercise are so important. Much of this weight gain is the result of a slowing metabolism. The following statistics tell the story:

◆ **Body weight:** 90 per cent of menopausal women gain an average of 5.4kg (12lb).

◆ **Metabolism:** The metabolism of a menopausal woman typically decreases by 10 to 15 per cent. (If you typically take in 1800 calories per day, a slowing metabolism would mean you would gain weight unless you reduced your average daily intake to 1620 calories per day.)

◆ **Percentage of body fat:** This figure may increase by one to four per cent.

◆ **Upper-body fat:** The increased ratio of testosterone to oestrogen at menopause typically increases a woman's waist-to-hip ratio from 0.75 to 0.95. (To calculate waist-to-hip ratio, divide your waistline in centimetres/inches by your hip measurement in centimetres/inches.)

Soya products, by the way, can actually decrease a man's risk of developing prostate cancer and even slow the growth of the disease in men who have it. And green vegetables are one of several good sources of a nutrient that is particularly important for the elderly: folate. A B-vitamin that is also found in pulses, citrus fruits, tomatoes, almonds, whole-wheat bread, bananas and cantaloupe melons – as well as in spinach, romaine lettuce, broccoli and other green vegetables – folate is necessary to regulate your body's level of homocysteine. What is homocysteine and why should it be regulated? It is an amino acid produced in the body, and studies have shown that too much of it in the blood can put you at higher risk of coronary heart disease, stroke and blood clots. The way people today worry about cholesterol is the way they should worry about homocysteine. According to experts, homocysteine, which causes fat deposits along the artery walls, may be more dangerous.

BE A FAN OF FOLATE

Folate – and its supplement form, folic acid – keeps the level of homocysteine down. The amount of folic acid suggested for regulating homocysteine is 400 micrograms (µg) per day. Typically, most one-a-day multivitamins contain 200µg – and I recommend that everyone take a multivitamin every day.

Whether you take multivitamins or not, the best way to get folic acid is in food, and green vegetables or beans are prime sources. For example, 230g of cooked spinach contains 265µg, and 230g of cooked white beans 250µg. In the UK, Australia and New Zealand, the Reference Nutrient Intake (RNI) of folic acid for men and women is just 200µg, so you can see how much of a punch a serving of vegetables packs.

The best idea of all is to cut back on dairy and meat, try soya substitutes and pulses, and eat as many fruits and vegetables – cooked, canned, raw, in soup – as you can.

In fact, the eating principles of Picture Perfect Weight Loss are absolutely picture

> **I recommend that everyone take a daily multivitamin**

perfect for the needs of older people. With its emphasis on fruit and vegetables; its focus on pulses, seafood and soya products for protein; and its goal of keeping the calorie count and saturated-fat content low and the enjoyment factor high, this plan is just right for an age group that needs lots of nutrients and energy without weight gain.

Of course, older people should check with their doctors about any food restrictions or food requirements they might have – but then, that's true of anyone at any age.

EXERCISE FOR OLDER PEOPLE

At the same time that older people are taking in the nutrients of a balanced, sensible, low-calorie diet, it's also extremely important that they exercise. Regular exercise on a permanent basis can actually help prevent disabilities and diseases such as heart ailments, diabetes and some types of cancer. The questions are obvious: what kind of exercise should you do and how much?

Check with your doctor before starting any exercise programme, but once you get the go-

> ### Learn a sport you've always wanted to learn

ahead, it's important to commit to a regular schedule. Every day of the week, if possible – certainly most days of the week – get at least 30 minutes of sustained, moderate physical activity, the kind of physical activity that makes you breathe harder. This kind of rhythmic, aerobic effort is calculated to build up your stamina. If you can't put in 30 minutes all at once, try three 10-minute sessions. But make sure you do a total of 30 minutes during the day, and make sure that each 10-minute session leaves you at least a little breathless.

How breathless? Here's a useful formula: if you can talk without any trouble at all, your exercise activity is too easy. If you can't talk at all, it's too hard. During a brisk walk, you should be able to carry on a conversation with a companion, but you'll be puffing what you say rather than speaking it.

Walking is one of the best endurance activities there is; it's good for the heart, leg muscles and overall trimness. It's also an exercise you can do anywhere, and it doesn't cost a thing.

But walking isn't the only endurance exercise for older people. Cycling is also excellent. So is dancing. So is doing a sport you've always loved to do – or learning a sport you've always wanted to learn. Swimming, tennis, badminton: all keep you on the move in a sustained way over time.

MAINTAINING MUSCLE MASS

In addition to endurance, you'll need to exercise your muscles. The ageing process does result in loss of muscle mass – and thus of physical strength. But the main reason for muscle loss over time is that many older people stop doing everyday activities that require strength. The solution? Don't stop doing such activities. In fact, go out of your way to undertake them. Do the household chores. Mow the grass. Rake the leaves. Begin

PHYTOCHEMICALS FIGHT CANCER

Red, yellow, orange: the colours of fruit and vegetables aren't just beautiful, they're beneficial to your lungs as well.

Yellow and orange fruit and vegetables are full of carotenoids and alpha-carotene, which may help reduce the risk of lung cancer. Red lycopene, which gives tomatoes their colour, is beneficial even to smokers, so now there's an even better reason to tuck into pasta, salads, tomato juice – even pizza!

You won't get the same benefits from taking pills or supplements though; it's the way the phytochemical compounds work together in foods that makes the difference. What's more, they also fight other cancers and heart disease as well.

SALT: WHAT'S THE STORY?

Where weight loss is concerned, salt, which contains no calories, is negligible. While the amount of salt in your diet might influence the amount of fluid in your body, it will have no effect whatsoever on you losing or gaining fat.

If your doctor has limited your intake of salt, it is probably for reasons of high blood pressure or hypertension. In this case, there are still plenty of alternatives for flavouring your food: a range of tinned tomato products for making sauces, for example, and just about anything with a tart or sweet-and-sour flavour. In addition, as the contents of your supermarket shelves demonstrate, a lot of soups and sauces are available in low-sodium versions; enhance their flavouring with lemon juice, herbs and spices, vinegars, horseradish or even wine.

But here's an important point to consider: if you've been advised to limit your salt intake because of high blood pressure and you're overweight, the Picture Perfect Weight Loss programme is probably the best eating plan you can follow. Eat the Picture Perfect Weight Loss pyramid (*see page 57*) and exercise routinely; you will soon lose weight and, in turn, help lower your blood pressure.

a more or less formal programme of resistance training focusing on low-impact weight-bearing exercise. Menopausal women in particular can benefit from such exercise, since bone density is a serious concern once they've stopped producing oestrogen. Yes,

The ageing process results in loss of muscle mass

such exercise can certainly include lifting light weights. The benefits are worth it: strong leg and hip muscles support you better, making it less likely that you'll fall. And strong muscles may contribute to bone strength as well.

Balance is another thing you can improve through weight-bearing exercise, and also by doing exercises like tai chi and yoga. Tai chi is based on Chinese Taoist philosophy and focuses on principles of yielding, softness, slowness, balance and suppleness. It is graceful, slow and a boon to balance. It requires no particular skill, demands no particular proficiency.

Yoga, another ancient form of exercise postures – from India this time – helps you shape up as it teaches you to chill out. Yoga can be particularly helpful for people with arthritis; it also helps relieve or manage stress, improve muscle tone, build strength and stamina, and improve circulation. Yoga keeps people incredibly supple – and strong – no matter what their age.

In fact, stretches of all types are increasingly important the older we get. The range of motion that stretching increases is extremely important in keeping the body's joints supple and 'well-oiled'. So keep moving. One way or another, push your body's limits just a little bit each day. Remember: if you keep on doing it, you find that you *can* keep on doing it. It's half the weight-loss battle – and it will keep you feeling young.

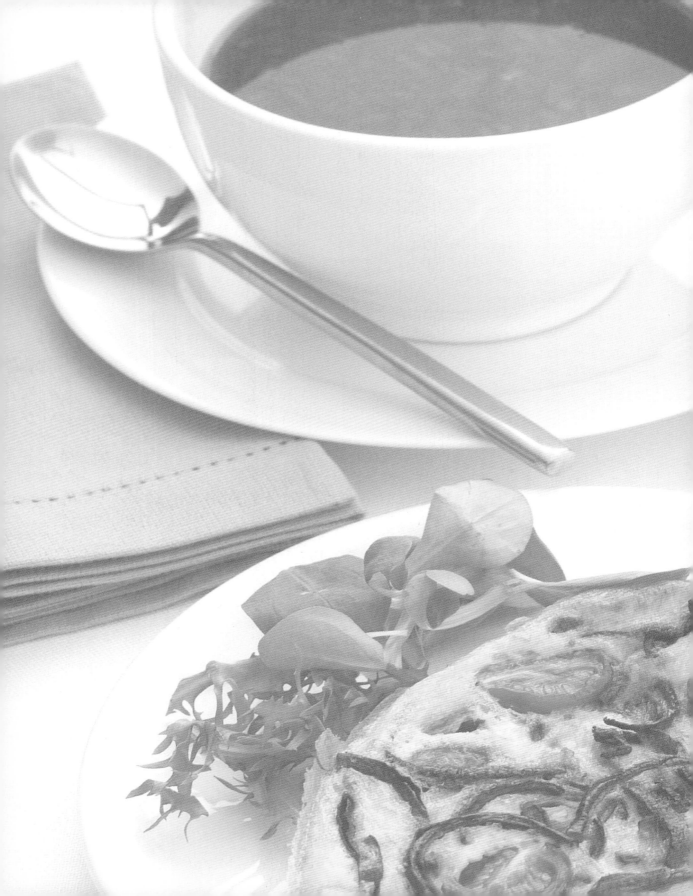

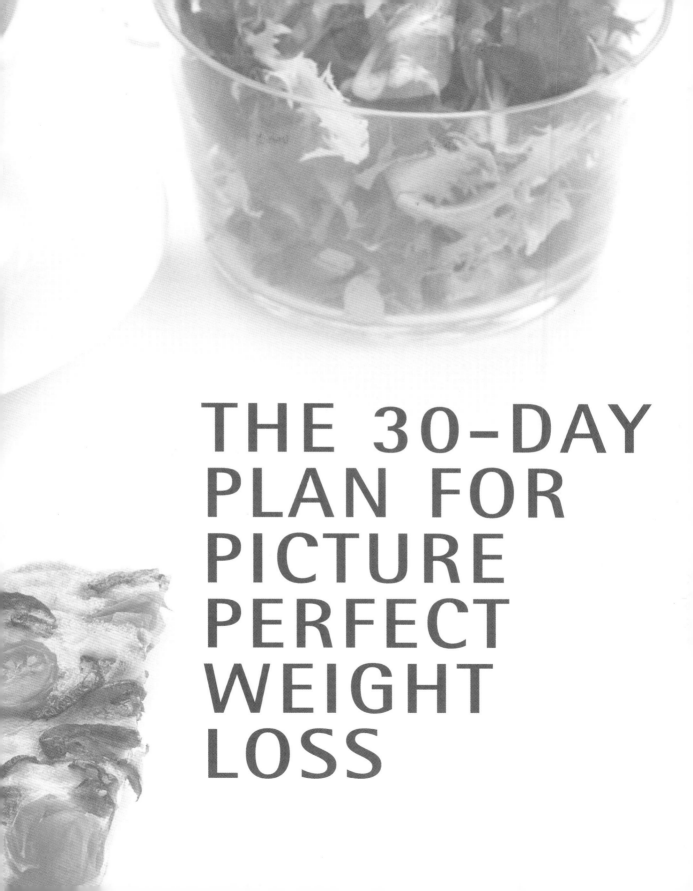

THE 30-DAY PLAN FOR PICTURE PERFECT WEIGHT LOSS

CHAPTER 3: DAY 1 – LET'S GO SHOPPING

YOUR DAY 1 AGENDA

By the end of Day 1, you will have:
◆ *Really* learned to read nutrition labels.
◆ Understood how supermarkets work.
◆ Changed the foods in your fridge, freezer and larder.
◆ Taken the first, empowering step towards Picture Perfect Weight Loss.

Today is Day 1 of changing your relationship with food – the one certain way to finally lose the weight you want to lose and keep it off. But where do you start to change your relationship with food? The answer is simple. You start in the supermarket. Or at the local deli. Or the farmer's market. Or the corner shop. Or wherever you buy the food you and your family will eat.

After all, choosing the food you'll buy is the first step in the process of eating. So to change your eating habits, you must first change your

> ## Calorie reduction is the key to weight loss

food-shopping choices. Think of the supermarket as your first opportunity to make the kinds of low-calorie choices pictured throughout this book. Every food-shopping trip is an occasion for you to assert that you've taken control, and that weight loss is your choice for life.

This chapter will offer some shopping guidelines to help you. I'll present my Anytime List (*see page 51*). Make it your own personal shopping list, and you'll be well on your way towards Picture Perfect Weight Loss for life. In addition, through the pages of this book, I'll walk the aisles of the supermarket with you to offer some suggestions on what foods to look for.

FOOD AWARENESS TRAINING: A REVIEW

First, let's review the principles of FAT – Food Awareness Training – that you were first introduced to in Chapter 1.

Principle One states that calorie reduction is the key to weight loss. Picture Perfect

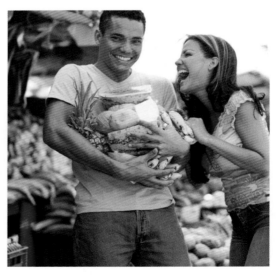

Groceries for goodness
Picture Perfect Weight Loss makes shopping fun, and encourages you to try as many new foods as possible.

Weight Loss happens when you are comfortable choosing low-calorie foods instead of high-calorie foods. Therefore, when shopping for food, you need to make a conscious effort to look for, find and buy the lower-calorie options that you like.

There are no forbidden foods in Picture Perfect Weight Loss

Principle Two of Food Awareness Training states that choice doesn't mean deprivation. This is because deprivation is counter-productive and can actually lead to weight *gain* rather than weight loss. That's why there are no forbidden foods in Picture Perfect Weight Loss, and it's why I stress that food is not your enemy. Nor is there any such thing as a 'correct' portion or an 'incorrect' reason for eating. When you want to eat, do so – and eat till you're satisfied.

This doesn't mean, though, that you can lose weight without making changes in your food choices. On the contrary, Picture Perfect Weight Loss asks you to stop doing what you've done and do something different, to make some fundamental changes. With Picture Perfect Weight Loss, however, you have the tools to make changes without condemning yourself to a restrictive diet and to the guilt – even the self-loathing – that tends to happen with such limited regimes.

Principle Three says that you can achieve Picture Perfect Weight Loss while living your life. In fact, I insist on it. Hold a lavish dinner party, head for the fridge when you need a break from housework, take your clients out to lunch, travel five days of the week – whatever your life is, whatever your tastes are, Picture Perfect Weight Loss lets you accommodate them comfortably. Through

Food Awareness Training, you can make the choices that will lead to Picture Perfect Weight Loss without causing your own personal world to stop turning.

Remember: you are not on a diet. Instead, you're involved in a lifelong process of making healthy, low-calorie choices at every meal, in every eating situation and whenever and wherever you shop for food.

Put these three principles together and you have a pretty straightforward guide to shopping for Picture Perfect Weight Loss:
■ You'll be looking for low-calorie choices every time you food shop.
■ You'll be embracing a wider range of choices – including some foods you've never tried before.
■ You'll be shopping for foods you enjoy – foods that suit your taste and your lifestyle.

MORE FOR LESS: MORE FOODS FOR LESS WEIGHT

Once inside the doors of your supermarket – or wherever you shop – remind yourself of this: you're not giving up the foods you love; rather, you're adding to your life more foods that you're going to love just as much. You're seeking alternatives, not necessarily replacements. You're trying to extend your options, not narrow them. You're going to lose weight, and in doing so you're going to gain health, well-being, a better appearance and a way of eating you can live with and enjoy for a lifetime.

For a chocolate lover, for example, there's no such thing as a substitute for chocolate – but there may be new ways to get your chocolate that reduce the calorie impact, and there are certainly other options for satisfying that sweet tooth. Or maybe you're a meat-and-potatoes guy. Strange as it may sound, there really is a whole range of low-calorie

FIGURING OUT FOOD NUTRITION LABELS

Food nutrition labels are a great information source. They're the 'study guide' to a lot of the foods that you're eating, and you'll find them on most food packages these days. But what can you do with the label information?

Knowing what it says on the nutrition information label isn't much good by itself. That's especially the case for people on my programme, because Food Awareness Training does not entail calorie-counting, portion-weighing or nutrient-measuring.

There's no magic number of calories you should or should not eat every day, and no special serving size that will enable you to lose weight. I won't even tell you to eat a certain combination of nutrients that will produce the desired results.

On the other hand, this information is worth knowing. By reading the nutrition information label carefully, you can quickly learn how much of certain nutrients the food contains – paying particular attention to the 'bad guys' such as saturated fat.

To get the most from a food label, you have to read it correctly. Start with the serving size. It's the basis for all the other facts and figures on the label.

Once you've read the serving size, take a moment to think about what you really eat, and compare that to the serving size described on the label. On a jar of olives, the label might indicate that three olives is the serving size, but if you usually eat six, you need to double the calories and all other nutritional figures to find out what you're actually getting when you eat those half-dozen olives.

Government regulations on what information is compulsory on food labelling vary from country to country. In some cases, only the energy value, amount of protein, carbohydrate and fat per 100g or 100ml need be given; for others, the amounts of saturated fat, sugar, dietary fibre and sodium is also required.

If a claim is made about the food – for example, that it is low-fat or contains certain vitamins or minerals – the quantities of these must also be included on the label.

The following definitions apply in the UK to the use of certain claims on food packaging:
◆ A low-calorie food should have 40 calories (167kJ) or fewer per serving. A low-calorie soft drink must have 10 calories (42 kJ) or fewer per 100ml.
◆ A low-fat food should have 3g or less of fat per 100g or 100ml.
◆ A food that has low saturated fat contains 1.5g or less of saturated fat per 100g or 100ml.
◆ A low-sodium food should have 40mg or less of sodium per 100g or 100ml.
◆ A reduced-energy food should have no more than three quarters of the energy value of a comparable food.

However, these guidelines are only recommendations rather than law in many countries. Your best bet is to look at the label, compare it with other foods, and work out for yourself whether it is a good choice or not.

Understanding the data on the label makes you a more informed shopper and a more thoughtful eater. That's reason enough to browse the nutrition labels when you're making your selections at the supermarket.

alternatives that are just as tasty as meat and potatoes and will more than satisfy your palate. You just haven't found them yet.

Your weekly or daily shopping trip is your chance to be both thoughtful and creative about changing your relationship with food. The chapters that follow will expand your thinking and stir your creativity with ideas and suggestions that focus on specific meals, one week at a time. And the food demonstrations that you will see throughout this book will serve as an encyclopedia of possible choices – and a reference tool you can go back to again and again. But it's *your* tastes, *your* preferences and *your* imagination that will really make the difference. As I've said before in this book and will say again: your Picture Perfect Weight Loss is in your hands. With that in mind, let's go shopping.

LOOK AND LEARN

I call my weight-loss programme *Picture Perfect* Weight Loss for a reason. Choosing begins in awareness, and awareness begins with seeing. In any supermarket you will see an almost dizzying array of choices.

Fortunately, today's foods offer a key awareness tool: the nutrition label. Once you know how to read it, it can be a useful guide to making low-calorie choices. Policewoman Dorothy Jackson recalls that the first time she went shopping using the principles of Picture Perfect Weight Loss, she spent four hours in the supermarket reading every word of every label of every food she was thinking about buying – and making choices based on what the labels told her. Dorothy's husband gave up and went to wait in the car. That was six years ago, before she lost the 22.6kg (50lb) she shed in six months of Picture Perfect Weight Loss eating and has kept off ever since. Now, she doesn't have to read labels; she has been a

Picture Perfect shopper for so long that she knows exactly what she's doing, and shopping for low-calorie, healthy, nutritious foods is second nature to her.

THREE KEY SHOPPING TIPS

I want to offer three key thoughts on shopping for Picture Perfect Weight Loss. Simply put, think variety, taste-enhancers – spices, garnishes, herbs, sauces, condiments of every sort – and soup. All are powerful tools in your weight-loss programme.

1. AVOID BOREDOM

Why is variety important to weight loss? Because boredom is tantamount to deprivation, and deprivation, as we know, is extremely detrimental to losing weight and keeping it off.

Is there any such thing as a diet that isn't boring? Fad diets often restrict people to just one food – for example, nothing but grapefruit, or only protein for breakfast and dinner and only carbohydrates for lunch. Other diets set up a daily, weekly or even monthly menu. Your entire eating future is laid out for you. There are no surprises, there's no room to add the foods you find appetising – or even the food you just

Fad diets often restrict people to just one food

suddenly 'feel like' eating right this minute for no apparent reason. Boredom denies your natural appetite, and restrictive diets eventually fail for just that reason.

In fact, the boredom doesn't just prompt people to go off the fad diet or disobey the daily menu; it can actually cause weight gain. Why? Because boring eating is work; it's drudgery. And if you've put up with drudgery for a few days, or for a week, or for more, then you deserve something delicious as compensation. Or so you tell yourself – in what easily becomes a convincing argument. The consequence, however, is that you end up eating a rich, high-calorie meal or meals as a 'reward' for the work of eating all that bland, tasteless food.

So how do you avoid boredom? Never was there a better time to try new foods and expand your tastes than when you are undertaking the Picture Perfect Weight Loss programme. Let's face it: far too many of us

Broaden your culinary horizon and widen your vision

are stuck with a limited food vocabulary. We know what we like, and we tend not to stray too far from what we know. So protein means meat or dairy, a salad consists of iceberg lettuce, vegetables equal potatoes, and dessert is chocolate cake. Full stop.

Okay, you may know what you like, but there is a vast universe of foods out there, and

it probably includes foods you will come to enjoy. In fact, there might be something out there you'll like even more than what you're eating now. Without exception, every one of my patients has told me how Picture Perfect Weight Loss introduced him or her to new taste sensations. From the firefighters who found they love veggie burgers . . . to the priest who once thought seafood meant fish sticks and now knows it includes salmon, tuna and lobster . . . to the lawyer who 'discovered' pulses at the age of 45 – whole new worlds of taste, texture and nourishment can open up to you, if you let them.

Try something you've never tried before. If you don't like it, don't eat it again – but at least try it. It will make your weight-loss programme easier – and a lot more fun. For example, in addition to the fish you've been used to since childhood, how about trying some variations on the theme – smoked

Fruits to suit
It's now possible for us to buy a huge variety of fruit from around the world – and they are all available at your local supermarket.

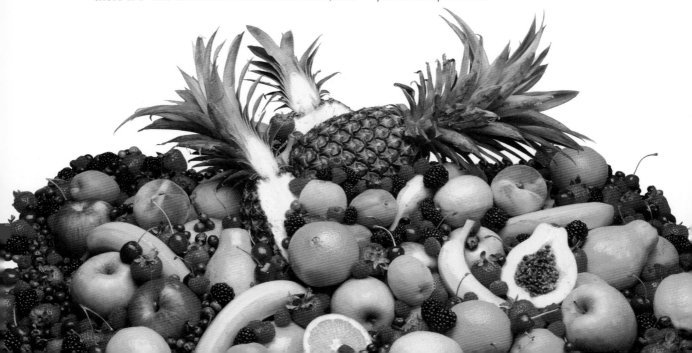

UNDISCOVERED VEGETABLES: MAKE NEW FRIENDS

Picture yourself in your supermarket's produce section. The apples are on your left, right next to the oranges. On your right are the celery, cucumbers and carrots. In the middle, as though they can't quite decide if they're fruit or vegetables, reside the tomatoes. Next time you're at the supermarket, take a closer look. I bet that interspersed among the green lettuce, yellow peppers and red tomatoes are vegetables you've never noticed. Just as strangers are friends you haven't met yet, some of those unfamiliar vegetables could be your new favourites, just waiting to be discovered. Here are a few ideas:

◆ Artichokes aren't nearly as difficult to eat as their spiny shape suggests. Members of the sunflower family, artichokes originated in Sicily. Choose tightly furled artichokes – the fatter the better. The tender bases of the petals and the fleshy heart to which the petals are connected are the parts you can eat. You can boil, steam or microwave them and serve them in stews, salads and casseroles.

◆ Bok choy, or pak choi, has crunchy white stalks and mild-tasting, tender, dark green leaves. It can be eaten raw, but it is usually cooked. It's often used as an ingredient in stir-fries and Oriental-style soups.

◆ Bean sprouts are the tender young sprouts from the mung bean. You should use only the freshest, white-looking sprouts. They can be eaten raw in salads or cooked slightly in stir-fries to keep their light and crisp qualities. Keep them in the fridge for up to three days.

◆ Watercress is a vegetable with a long history. Persian, Greek and Roman soldiers ate this leafy vegetable to prevent scurvy during their military campaigns. This member of the mustard family grows in cool running water. Its pungent flavour is slightly bitter, with a peppery snap. Try it cooked, tossed in salads or as a great way to add a crunch to sandwiches.

salmon, for instance . . . or canned sardines or kippers or smoked mackerel or smoked oysters . . . maybe smoked trout? Your eyes have probably just passed over these items on the supermarket shelves in the past. Try them.

If your idea of condiments stops at bright red ketchup, dreary brown sauce and garish yellow mustard, it's time to move on – to Caribbean jerk sauce, sweet-and-sour sauce, mint sauce, an endless range of barbecue and grilling marinades, and such pepper-hot sauces as Tabasco and jalapeño, to name just a couple. There are also mustards that are stone-ground, flavoured or created in specific regions, such as Dijon.

Even fruit, of which we have an abundance in the western world, has recently enjoyed a culinary franchise expansion. It isn't just pears and apples anymore – Conference and Granny Smiths – now you can find scores of varieties of the common fruits. In addition, there are the relatively uncommon fruits: mango, papaya, apricots, a range of melons in every colour – from Piel de Sapo to Orange Flesh to Juan Canary to Galia melon from Israel and carillon melon from France, figs, kumquats, kiwi fruit, nectarines, green and red and white and black grapes, clementines, pomegranates, berries of every shape and hue, and tropical fruits such as passion fruit, pomelo and custard apple. Try them all. In fact, why not try a new fruit every week for the next few weeks?

The bottom line? Broaden your culinary horizon and widen your vision. There's a world of food out there. You'll appreciate Picture Perfect Weight Loss even more when you experience the richness of the world's foods in all their diverse colours, textures and tastes – available today in your local supermarket.

2. SPICE UP YOUR LIFE

Variety is essential to Picture Perfect Weight Loss. After all, variety is the spice of life. And spicing up your meals is important to Picture Perfect Weight Loss and to shopping for Picture Perfect Weight Loss.

Buy loads of taste-enhancers, such as spices, garnishes, herbs, sauces and condiments. Why?

> ## Load your shopping trolley with low-fat condiments

Because they add taste, flavour and more creativity to your cooking and eating. Add some basil to a salad dressing . . . enliven a soup with freshly ground black pepper . . . season your vegetable dip with Thai curry paste. The time is right to experiment with recipes, especially as you're about to extend the range of your food choices. A well-stocked shelf of flavourings will help your trial-and-error process and give you more options. And options, in a very real sense, are what Picture Perfect Weight Loss is all about.

3. SOUP THINGS UP

Soups are another powerful tool of weight loss. The groups of firefighters I've worked with are particularly big soup fans, and many have become highly creative soup chefs. A bowl of hearty soup can be an entire meal. It's also a great way to eat your vegetables – even if you're someone who isn't a big fan of vegetables. Plus, you can use soups in other recipes – as a marinade, for example, or to create a sauce.

DR SHAPIRO'S ANYTIME LIST

You can probably guess how the Anytime List got its name: where Picture Perfect Weight Loss is concerned, anything on the list is good to eat at any time, in any amount, for any purpose, driven by any motivation. Keep these foods on hand to eat either as a snack or as part of a meal. Make vegetables, fruit and the lowest-calorie frozen sweets and desserts the core of your eating, and you stand a superb chance of being thin for life – just by eating foods you *want* to eat.

Load your shopping trolley with low-fat condiments of every variety to give your food extra flavour. Enjoying your food is essential for both weight loss and a lifetime of weight control. Then head for the frozen food aisle. If you're the type of person who needs a quick meal occasionally, you may wish to toss a few frozen low-calorie meals into your shopping trolley, along with a generous supply of frozen vegetables and fruit. Above all, don't forget frozen seafood.

Also stock up on a good range of drinks. There is a profusion of low-calorie hot chocolates available. Most range from 20 to 50 calories per packet (it's best to avoid hot drinks that carry more than that). Check the labels – avoid drinks labelled 'naturally sweetened' or 'fruit-juice sweetened', since they tend to be full of calories.

Once your cupboards and freezer are crammed with the basics, going shopping becomes pretty much a matter of buying the fresh foods that complete the meal.

DR SHAPIRO'S ANYTIME LIST

The following foods are the best bets for any time of year. If you have these foods at the ready, they'll be the first that you reach for when you're hungry. So here's my prescription for the foods that you should keep on hand.

VEGETABLES
All kinds of vegetables – raw, cooked, fresh, frozen, tinned or in soups.

FRUIT
All fruit – raw or cooked, fresh, frozen or tinned. (Avoid any packaged fruit with added sugar.)

DRINKS
Help yourself to any low-calorie drinks. Ones to keep in stock include:

Coffees and teas Including fruit and herbal teas and iced tea and coffee
Diet fizzy drinks Any preference of flavours
Instant hot chocolate Look for mixes that have 20 to 50 calories per serving. Avoid cocoa mixes that have 60 calories or more
Milkshake mixes You want the kinds that have 70 or fewer calories per serving

FROZEN DESSERTS
All kinds of fat-free frozen yoghurt, sorbet or ice lollies are good to have in your freezer. When selecting brands, be sure to keep an eye on the calories.

SWEETS
Chewing gum
Hard-boiled sweets Such as lollipops, rock, humbugs and butterscotch

CONDIMENTS AND SEASONINGS
All the flavourful ingredients listed below are low-calorie. Use them creatively to spice up your vegetable courses, treats and snacks.

Oil-free or low-calorie salad dressings
Fat-free or low-fat mayonnaise, low-fat crème fraîche
Fat-free yoghurt Natural or artificially sweetened
Mustards Dijon and other kinds
Tomato Purée, passata, tomato juice
Lemon or lime juice
Oil sprays In butter or olive-oil flavours
Vinegars Balsamic, cider, tarragon, wine or other flavours
Sauces Barbecue, chutney, ketchup, relish, salsa, soy, tamari, Worcestershire, hoisin, horseradish, miso, black bean and oyster
Onion Fresh, flakes or powder
Garlic Fresh, purée, flakes or powder
Herbs All kinds, including basil, bay leaves, chives, dill, oregano, rosemary, sage, tarragon and thyme
Spices All kinds, including allspice, cinnamon, cloves, coriander, cumin, curry powder, ginger, nutmeg, paprika and pepper
Extracts Including almond, coconut, peppermint and vanilla
Cocoa powder
Stock cubes

PACKAGE DEAL

One more word as you prepare to head out the door for the supermarket: don't ignore tinned, packaged or frozen foods. I know that some people believe there's a tendency to think that fruit and vegetables must be fresh to be good. This isn't necessarily so.

Don't get me wrong. I think fresh fruit and vegetables are the best foods on the planet – for health, weight loss and sheer goodness. But the fact is that the goodness, the weight-loss potential and the health benefits of fruit and vegetables are often just as powerful in packaged form as in the fruit and vegetables that were fresh-picked this morning. Did you know that fruit and vegetables intended for packaging are typically harvested at their absolute peak of freshness? That freshness is preserved by the packaging, whatever its form. And while it is true that the processing required to preserve a food can sometimes cause the loss of nutrients, it is also true that the loss is tiny – almost infinitesimal.

Besides, the loss is more than offset by the benefits that packaging provides. What are those benefits? For one thing, the technology behind preservation means that you can enjoy fruit and vegetables out of season, even all year long. Summer fruits throughout the winter . . . autumn vegetables in the spring. This luxurious health benefit would have astonished preceding generations.

SHOPPING FOR YOUR KIDS

At just around your waist level as you push your trolley around the supermarket aisles – at eye level for your kids – are the products made especially to appeal to children. As a parent, you need to be very wary of these foods pitched at kids. While many are suitable choices, in terms of both calorie count and nutrition, others are high-calorie products with little nutritional value, if any.

The latter food choices confirm my key recommendation about shopping for children who may be overweight. It's this: shopping for kids is like shopping for yourself. The same principles that guide you in buying supplies for your Picture Perfect Weight Loss should guide you in buying the foods for your children's Picture Perfect Weight Loss.

Pay particular attention to snack foods. Growing children do snack, of course, and snack-food manufacturers make no secret of the fact that they are targeting young people. If your child is overweight, be especially careful about snack foods that *sound like* they're weight-conscious choices – dietetic sweets, for example, or all-natural crisps. As the demonstrations show, some of these can be what I call saboteur foods – you buy into the advertising claim that this is a weight- or health-conscious choice, so you eat even more of the snack than you might have if it were not 'dietetic', only to find out that the calorie saving isn't that great, if it exists at all, and the nutritional value is low.

Expand your scope of food options, not just for yourself, but for your children too. Remember: no child should feel deprived of the tastes he or she enjoys, but by expanding choices, you can also expand the range of your child's enjoyment. More varieties of foods mean more nutritional benefits.

SALTY SNACKS

If you're craving a salty snack but are concerned about the high calorie count of peanuts, try roasted soya nuts. You'll find them in health food shops. Dry-roasted or oil-roasted – and available in a range of flavours – a handful of soya nuts has half the fat content of peanuts (although it's the healthier unsaturated fat in both cases) and considerably fewer calories. Soya nuts also provide folate and fibre, iron and other minerals, and disease-fighting isoflavones.

The convenience of tinned, packaged and frozen fruit and vegetables is another luxury. Think about it: any time of year, any time of day or night, just open a can or packet, and with minimal preparation you are ready to serve and eat pineapple from the tropics, beans from the Mediterranean, new potatoes from Egypt – all without leaving home. It certainly saves on the expense of having to travel overseas to sample these luxuries!

Fruit and vegetables are at the heart of Picture Perfect Weight Loss. Technology makes it possible to enjoy them in all their variety all the time – without limit. That's a boon to anyone trying to lose weight and keep it off for life.

MORE ESSENTIAL INGREDIENTS

Okay. Let's assume you've stocked your shelves and cupboards with the items on the Anytime List. Let's also assume that your fridge, freezer and larder are stuffed with fresh, frozen and canned fruit and vegetables. In other words, you have the core of Picture Perfect Weight Loss sitting in your kitchen. But you'll probably still need to shop for a few more essential items. Here are some tips

and recommendations on how to look at the choices with which you'll be presented. You should look to have a generous supply of these foods in your kitchen to help you follow the Picture Perfect Weight Loss programme.

CEREALS

Let's start with breakfast cereals. The choices here are staggering, so let me offer a general rule: go for wholegrain or high-fibre cereal, and if possible, look for cereals that contain bran. After that, the array of flavours and textures is your choice as you look for the lowest-calorie option. Be very careful to check the serving size when you're perusing the nutrition labels on cereal boxes. These vary dramatically from manufacturer to

Don't ignore tinned, packaged or frozen foods

manufacturer, product to product, so be aware of exactly what you're buying.

Cereal bars are becoming increasingly popular with people who skip breakfast or eat it on the move. However, replacing a nutritional breakfast with a substitute cereal bar could be bad for your health. The UK campaign group Food Commission says tests on 18 products showed that all of them were high in fats, sugars or both. Of the 18 breakfast bars tested, all had higher levels of sugar than nutritionists recommend for a healthy breakfast such as a bowl of cereal with semi-skimmed milk. Ten had higher fat levels. Yet many were marketed as wholesome and ideal for school lunchboxes.

Food Commission says breakfast sets you up for the day, improves your concentration and limits pre-lunch snacking. So reach for the cereal box in the morning – not cereal bars.

BREADS AND SPREADS

Afraid you'll have to give up bread for Picture Perfect Weight Loss? Not necessarily. I recommend that you look for the light breads now offered in some stores. These have around 40 to 45 calories per slice. What's more, the slices are normal size, not those wafer-thin slivers that turn to mush on contact with tuna salad. If you do choose regular bread, look for wholegrain, which is the preferable nutritional choice. Make sure the packaging says '100 per cent wholegrain'.

Bread has excellent nutritional benefits. It is a good carrier of iron, fibre and the

> ### Substitute ready-made light dressings for vegetable oils

B-complex vitamins. From the point of view of weight control, bread is also very satisfying and filling – a good 'comfort food'. But bread also tends to be high in carbohydrate calories. My recommendation is to look at bread as a low-priority food – far below vegetables, fruit, pulses and seafood in the hierarchy of best choices.

Where jams and other sweet spreads are concerned, the lower-sugar versions are best – 10 to 20 calories per tablespoon compared with the 30 to 40 in regular jams. And don't be misled by honey, a wonderfully 'natural' food that actually has a higher concentrate of sugar than sugar itself. With no particular health benefits and weighing in at 50 calories per tablespoon, honey is best avoided if weight loss is your aim.

What about peanut butter? It often gets a bad press, and yes, it *is* a high-calorie item. But it is also very good for you. Peanut butter contains lots of nutrients that are important for heart health – niacin, folate, phosphorus,

vitamin E and phytosterols. So eat it in moderation, but make sure you *do* eat it.

OILS AND DRESSINGS

Everyone knows that vegetable oils are good for you, but their 120 calories per tablespoon are a high price to pay for the goodness. For the weight-conscious, in particular, I recommend substituting ready-made light dressings for vegetable oils.

In addition to serving as a substitute for oil or butter, ready-made dressings are a great food preparation ingredient – and that makes them a highly useful tool in Picture Perfect Weight Loss. Brush an avocado with a low-calorie tomato and basil dressing, for example, or drizzle king prawns in low-calorie Italian dressing in preparation for the grill. Or mix up a ready-made dressing with some low-calorie salsa to create a healthy vegetable dip. Another tip for salad lovers trying to shed pounds: use a flavoured vinegar as a salad dressing (or as a cooking ingredient) and forget the oil altogether.

FROZEN MEALS

When convenience is an issue, frozen meals are an excellent option. For breakfast, lunch or dinner, they offer a range of choices –

> ### AVOCADOS? ABSOLUTELY!
>
> High in calories? Sort of. High in fat? Just the unsaturated kind – the kind you want to have. Furthermore, avocados are packed with potassium, beta-carotene, vitamin C and folate – and they're also a source of cholesterol-lowering sterols. A rich, tasty meal in itself, a single avocado offers about 170g (6 oz) of edible fruit. Like all fruit and vegetables, it's the best kind of food you can eat for healthy weight loss.

JUST JUICE?

We drink fruit juices because they're delicious, refreshing and (generally) packed with the essential vitamins we need every day. But soft-drink manufacturers have a lot to answer for – many are misleading shoppers over the high sugar levels in their juice drinks.

Often considered healthy alternatives to fizzy pop, many juice drinks contain less than 15 per cent fruit juice. Research carried out by *Which?* magazine showed some drinks contained up to six teaspoons of sugar, while others had a fruit juice content of as little as five per cent. Some manufacturers may be substituting sugar for real fruit, risking damage to our teeth.

Editor of *Which?* Graeme Jacobs said: 'All too often drinks fall short of the healthy image that helps sell them to well-meaning parents.'

Other ingredients of fruit juice drinks include vegetable oil, thickening agents and colours to make the drinks look like real fruit juice.

The solution? Choose *real* fruit to enjoy the *real* health benefits it has to offer.

including a variety of tastes and textures. Of course, you should shop for the lower-calorie choices; in general, they provide excellent nutritional value for the calories.

My one reservation concerns the small portion sizes of vegetables in most of the lunch and dinner frozen meals. Of course, there's a simple solution to this: just add a vegetable side dish or a salad to your frozen meal, or start off with a cup or bowl of vegetable-rich soup.

DRINKS

The rule of thumb here is to eat your calories rather than drink them. All juices, fizzy drinks and flavoured drinks are full of calories. Yet the soft drink you sip with a meal and the glass of orange juice you knock back for an afternoon pick-me-up are almost afterthoughts. Why spend precious calories on afterthoughts? Besides, if you're desperate for the taste of orange, you are far better off eating an orange: you'll get lots of vitamins

Eat your calories rather than drink them

and minerals, lots of fibre to fill you up, and about 45 calories – compared with a glass of orange juice containing about 100 calories.

You should also ensure you drink enough water. Water is essential for the growth and maintenance of our bodies, as it's involved in a number of biological processes. In adults, water comprises 50–70 per cent of our total body weight, and without fluid, our body's survival time is limited to a matter of days.

Many people do not consume enough water, and as a result may become dehydrated, experiencing symptons like headaches, tiredness and loss of concentration. In general, you should be looking to consume around 2.5 litres of water a day – with 1.8 litres obtained directly from drinks.

My advice is to buy water in bottles if you don't like the taste of tap water. Stick to diet drinks at all other times, and check out the other recommendations on the Anytime List.

> ## Think about relegating starchy grains to side-dish status

RICE, PASTA AND OTHER STARCHY GRAINS

Look for wholegrain varieties, which are more nutritious. While brown rice and wholewheat pasta are probably available in your supermarket, you may have to head for a health food store to find the more exotic varieties such as whole wheat couscous, bulgur wheat, barley and millet.

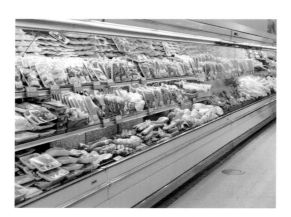

Supermarket savvy
The supermarket shelves are your gateway to Picture Perfect Weight Loss success. Learn how to navigate them and buy the foods that will benefit you most.

In general, as you stand in the supermarket aisle planning your meals in your mind, think about relegating the starchy grains to side-dish status. Fill up on vegetables and protein, and put rice, pasta, couscous and polenta in third place when you eat.

FROZEN DESSERTS

Look for low-fat, low-calorie ice cream, sorbet and yoghurt. But be certain to check the calorie counts; some products advertised as 'light' are nearly as high in calories as the real thing, making a mockery of the 'health' claim.

Fat-free frozen yoghurts and desserts are beginning to appear in supermarket chiller cabinets, but they are not to everyone's taste. If you cannot stomach fat-free frozen desserts, another option is low-fat desserts. These have the advantage of being available in a range of flavours to satisfy your dessert yearnings, but do go for the products with the lowest grams of fat per serving.

Enough shopping tips for one day? Okay, then check out the food demonstrations that appear over the following pages. After that, get to the supermarket and start buying!

YOUR DAY 1 GOALS

◆ Shop using the Anytime List.
◆ Buy four items you don't normally eat and try them. You may be pleasantly surprised, and you'll certainly be on your way to Picture Perfect Weight Loss.
◆ Buy a notebook. The next chapter will tell you why. Make sure it's small enough to carry with you during the day, but big enough to record everything you need to.
◆ Prepare to make changes.

THE PICTURE PERFECT WEIGHT LOSS FOOD PYRAMID

The Picture Perfect Weight Loss Food Pyramid is a guide to healthy, low-calorie choices. It maps the proportionate amounts of foods in an overall eating plan. Here's what it tells you.

Make fruit and vegetables the foundation of your eating. The pyramid is widest at the base, meaning you should let fruit and vegetables be the foods you eat most – most often, most regularly and most of.

Next, you should opt for protein. But as often as possible, get your protein from pulses and other legumes, seafood and soya rather than from meats, poultry and dairy products. When you take in grain products, try to choose wholegrain or 'light' versions.

Where fats and oils are concerned, you're looking to choose nuts, seeds, olives, avocados and olive oil wherever possible.

When you fancy something sweet, stick with hard-boiled sweets and either fat-free yoghurts or low-fat frozen desserts.

If you don't see your favourite food category on my pyramid, keep in mind that no food is forbidden with Picture Perfect Weight Loss. The pyramid presents my recommendations for a healthy way of eating that will provide all the nutrients you need as you lose weight and maintain your weight loss.

Make the Picture Perfect Weight Loss food pyramid your guide, and you will be thin for life.

Boiled sweets, fat-free yoghurt and low-fat frozen desserts
SWEETS

Nuts, seeds, olives, avocados, olive oil and other vegetable oils
FATS AND OILS

Preferably wholegrain or 'light' versions
GRAIN PRODUCTS

Preferably soya products, pulses and seafood
PROTEIN FOODS

Any and all - fresh, frozen, tinned, packaged - as much as possible, as often as possible
FRUIT AND VEGETABLES

OUR DAILY BREAD

Perhaps you've always eaten regular sliced white bread – at 80 to 90 calories per slice. Well why not try French bread at 50 calories per 2.5cm slice or – even better – light bread at just 40 to 45 calories per slice? All three equations may total 900 calories, but by eating light bread you'll get the most food for the fewest calories.

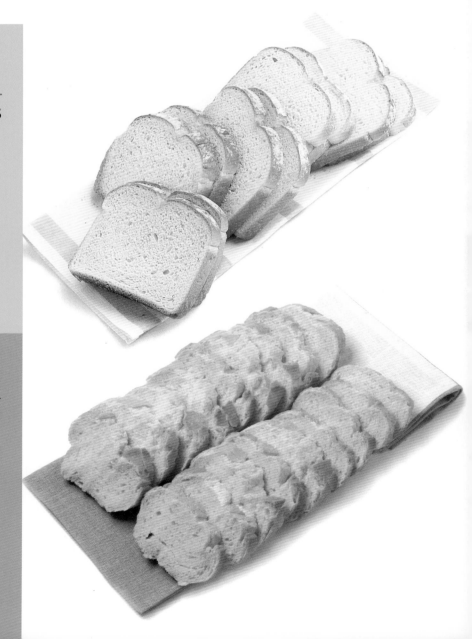

½ loaf regular bread
───────────────
900 calories

French bread
───────────────
900 calories

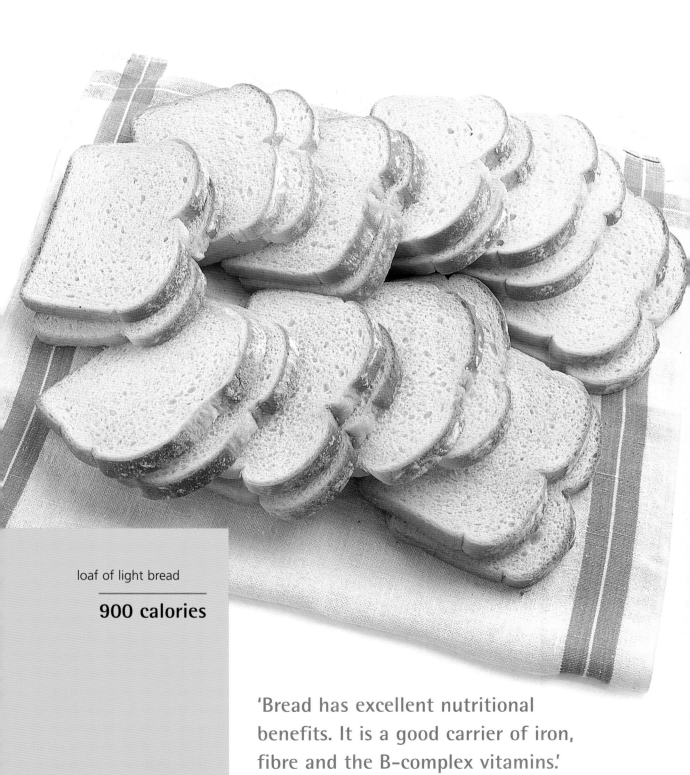

loaf of light bread

900 calories

'Bread has excellent nutritional benefits. It is a good carrier of iron, fibre and the B-complex vitamins.'

MILKING IT

Although I recommend only consuming milk in moderation, if you do drink it, bear in mind that not all types of milk have the same calorie content. My advice is to choose skimmed milk: you can drink twice as much as full-fat milk for the same calories. If you find skimmed milk too watery, however, try the semi-skimmed version – 380 calories' worth works out at 790ml.

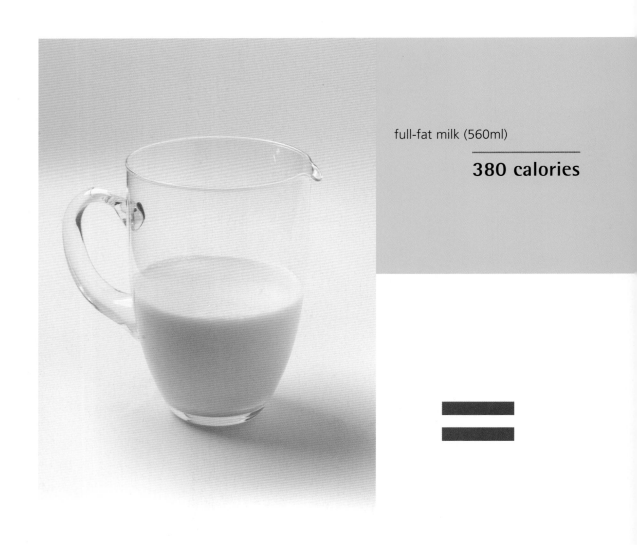

full-fat milk (560ml)

380 calories

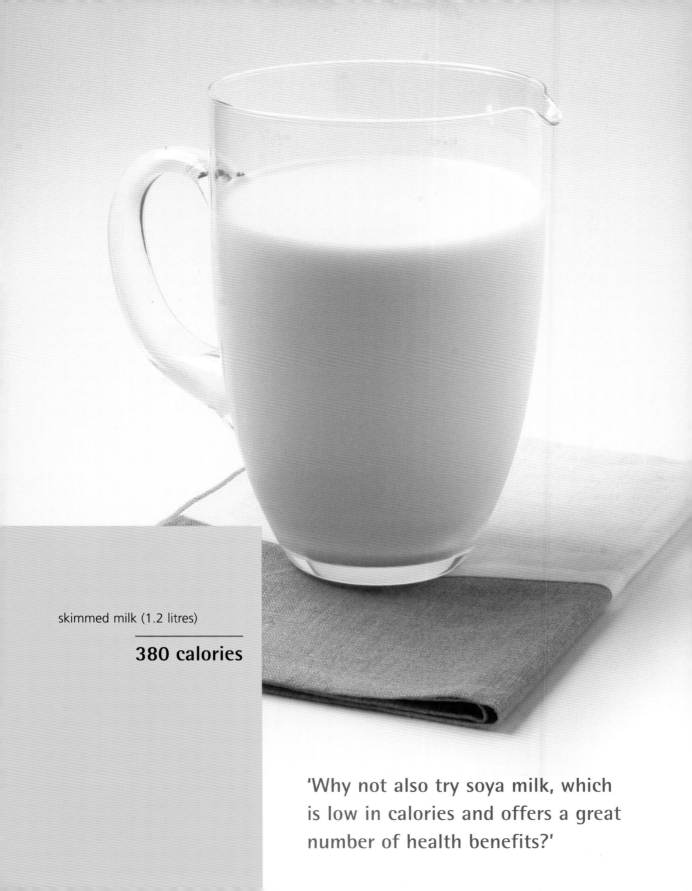

skimmed milk (1.2 litres)

380 calories

'Why not also try soya milk, which is low in calories and offers a great number of health benefits?'

BIN THE BUTTER

I always advocate using olive oil ahead of butter or margarine, especially as a cooking ingredient. But if you simply have to have some kind of spread on your toast, choose a low–fat spread. The taste isn't *that* different from butter, and you'll save yourself more than a whopping three times the calories.

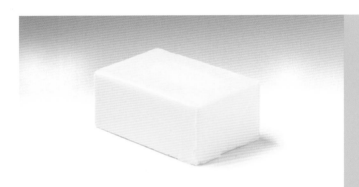

butter (250g)

1850 calories

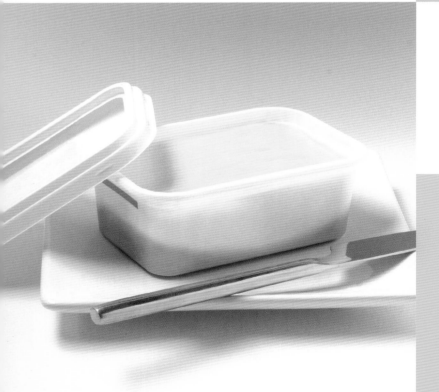

VS

low-fat spread (250g)

575 calories

PICK YOUR PÂTÉ CAREFULLY

A serving of pâté can make the perfect start to a meal – a little something to whet your appetite. But how much do you really want to whet it? The liver pâté below has a huge 450 calories per 100 grams, while the same amount of mushroom pâté contains almost two-thirds fewer calories at just 170.

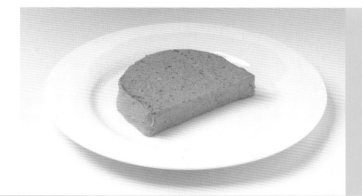

liver pâté (100g)
_____

450 calories

VS

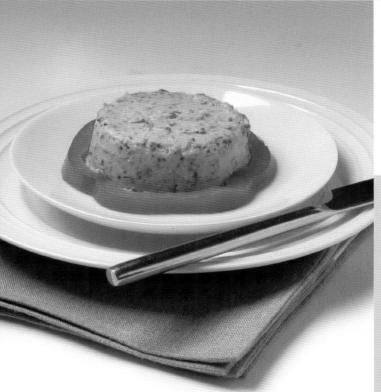

mushroom pâté (100g)
_____

170 calories

SORBET? YOU BET!

Luxury ice cream is delicious, I can't deny that, and we all enjoy tucking into a little bit of temptation occasionally. But this is a temptation that costs you – in calories. A serving of sorbet, however, has only half the calories of the ice cream. Look at the demonstration: twice the amount of food for the same number of calories. Now how refreshing is that?

'Sorbet is one of the foods featured on the Anytime List, so you can enjoy it at any time.'

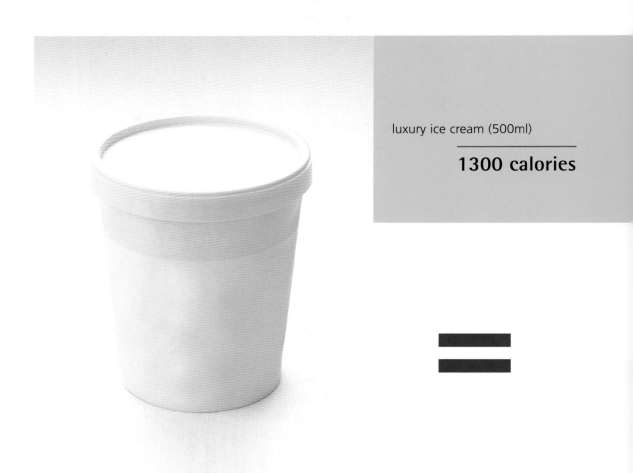

luxury ice cream (500ml)

1300 calories

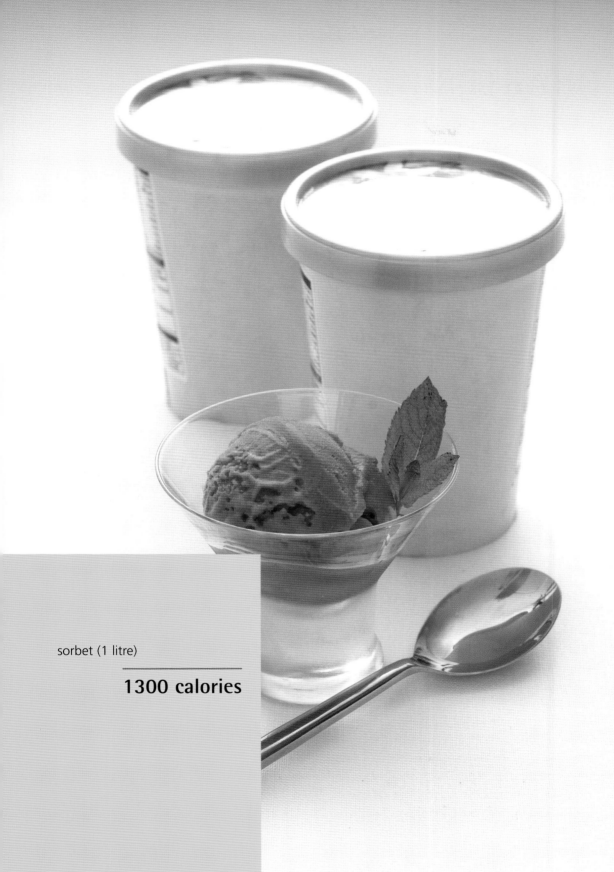

sorbet (1 litre)

1300 calories

CHAPTER 4: WEEK 1 – TIME TO FOCUS ON BREAKFAST

YOUR WEEK 1 AGENDA

By the end of Week 1, you will have:
◆ Committed to change.
◆ Learned the basic principles of Picture Perfect Weight Loss.
◆ Started a food diary/personal journal.
◆ Begun to exercise.
◆ Changed your thinking about breakfast and your breakfast choices.
◆ Begun to lose weight.

Week 1 of the 30-Day Plan for Picture Perfect Weight Loss is about more than just changing the way you think about your first meal of the day. It's actually about changing your life – by starting to change your relationship with food.

This is the moment when you begin forging the principles of Picture Perfect

You want to look better, feel better and live longer

Weight Loss, putting them in place so that they eventually become routine. That's an ambitious plan, but I make it doable by breaking it down into manageable steps. You're not going to change your relationship with food all at once, but rather one step at a time. Actually, for Week 1, I want you to undertake five specific steps. To start, get yourself a notebook. It will come in handy.

STEP 1: FOCUS ON YOUR MOTIVATION

Why are you doing this? Why are you starting today to undertake a programme of Picture Perfect Weight Loss – a programme that asks you to make a long-term, even lifetime commitment to change?

Of course, everybody knows the answer to this: you're doing it to lose weight. You want to look better, feel better, live longer. Everybody knows *all* the reasons why people try to lose weight.

But you're not 'people'. You're you. And the first step you should take towards Picture Perfect Weight Loss is to know the desire or need that is triggering you to undertake the programme – your personal motivation for changing your relationship with food.

Maybe the trigger for you, as for so many of the firefighters I've worked with, is suddenly feeling 'weighed down' by the extra weight you've accumulated – so much so, in the firefighters' case, that they wondered about their ability to do the job.

Maybe it's something as 'simple' as that forthcoming school reunion . . . or looking good in a bikini, not just this summer, but every summer in the future . . . or being tired of feeling different, left out, set apart from the world of thin people.

PUT IT DOWN ON PAPER

Whatever your personal motivation is, discover it, articulate it clearly, even say it out loud. Then write it down on its own page in your notebook so you can revisit it from time to time and channel your thoughts. Why is this important? Because if you don't understand clearly what motivates you, it's all too easy to lose focus. Especially at the very beginning of the programme, when everything is new and different, when Food Awareness has not yet become automatic and the principles of Picture Perfect Weight Loss

Writing things down is a 'focusing device'

have not yet become second nature, you will need to hold on tight to your motivating reason. You'll have to think in ways you haven't thought before, try foods you haven't tried before. You may feel uncomfortable in certain situations because change is often uncomfortable. Remembering exactly what weight loss can mean to you is probably the most powerful weapon you can have to keep you focused.

Make the notebook your workbook, your personal journal of the change you're going through, including any feelings of discomfort or things that are troubling you. Studies show that writing things down is a 'focusing device', as behaviourists call it, and what you're focusing on is your own power to make change, the importance of the change

PERFECT PRESENTATION

We eat with our eyes. Even the simplest of foods can become special when presented attractively. A touch of garnish, a beautiful serving dish, or a colourful arrangement all make food look so good that you *really* want to eat it. Try really focusing on presentation when you prepare your next meal.

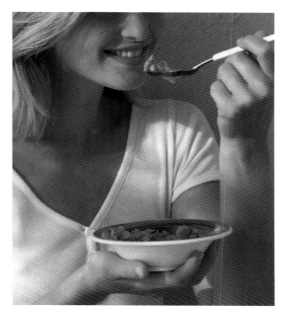

Breakfast of champions
Your first meal of the day is the first meal you'll change using the Picture Perfect Weight Loss programme – making food choices to set you up for the day ahead.

you're making, and the very personal need or desire that motivates you. Having these details written down will be useful to you.

FAILURE? FORGET IT

One more point about motivation. You've failed before? You've lost weight in the past, then regained it? Forget about it. Failure is an old and distant memory. Think of your past failures as rehearsals that didn't really count. Instead, fast-forward to today. Today is when change starts. From this moment forward, you're on the Picture Perfect Weight Loss programme, and all the signs are positive.

In fact, I recommend marking the moment in some way. When Tia and Jim Chisholm of the Chicago 7 embarked on Picture Perfect Weight Loss, they cleaned out their fridge and larder, getting rid of all the foods they decided should no longer be a part of their lives. Another patient of mine cancelled her newspaper delivery and decided instead to cycle or walk into town for the paper each morning. Because any kind of change can break a cycle, these gestures, while symbolic, mark the moment. They draw a line between one phase of your life – the one in which you were overweight – and the new you to come.

STEP 2: HONOUR THYSELF

A patient told me about the day she tried to begin her Picture Perfect Weight Loss programme. She was determined to start the day by getting on the exercise bike in the spare room and doing 10 minutes before breakfast. She had just sat on the saddle when her husband's voice boomed out from the kitchen, asking where the bread was. She got off the bike, went downstairs to show him it was in the bread bin (where it's always kept), and then returned to the bike. Not the most auspicious start, my patient thought.

Next it was her daughter who interrupted. She popped into the spare room, announced her after-school plans, and demanded her mother's undivided attention. My patient climbed off the bike and wrote this pertinent information on her list for the day.

Back on the bike. This time it was her son. He couldn't remember where he had put his hockey stick. Her husband again: was she going to cook breakfast? Daughter: just wondering if the dog had been fed. And so on. Later that morning, an elderly friend called needing a lift to the shops – could my patient drive her there?

The upshot of all this? My patient never did any exercise at all that day. She never found – never *took* – the 10 minutes she had promised herself. You have to. You have to do Picture Perfect Weight Loss for *you*. Sure, mothers are typically the pivotal figure in a family. They're the care providers, the hub around which the family moves. But everyone – even a small child – can wait 10 minutes while you do your exercise . . . or prepare a special meal . . . or take a relaxing bath . . . or go for a brisk walk. You deserve it.

Even if your motivating trigger is to be an example to your kids – in fact, *especially* if your motivating trigger is to be an example to your kids – set that example by caring for yourself as you want them to care for themselves.

> ## You have to do Picture Perfect Weight Loss for you

Stick a sign that says 'Honour Thyself' on your fridge or on the mirror in your bedroom. It's a reminder that where Picture Perfect Weight Loss is concerned, this one is for you. And don't get off the exercise bike until you've finished your routine. Your family will quickly get the idea that they need to request things from you before or after your exercise session.

SET UP A SUPPORT SYSTEM

To help you remember the importance of your weight-loss programme, try to set up your own support system. What do I mean by this? I mean someone who can help you hold on to your motivation, someone who will be comfortable with a different you. It might be a family member; it might be a friend. New York psychologist Adele Fink, whose practice is '75 per cent' focused on people with weight issues, talks about how unsettling a person's weight loss can be to family and friends. 'They're comfortable with the old you,' says Dr Fink. 'They want you to stay the same, and your weight loss – your change – can be threatening to them.'

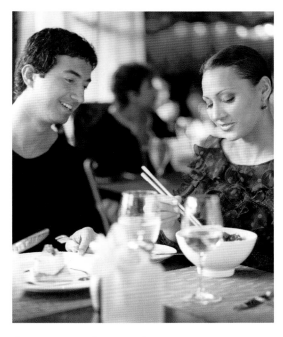

A message of support

You need to find someone – a friend, partner, relative or colleague – who will act as your 'support system' and encourage you in your new eating programme.

One patient told me about eating lunch with two friends. When she pulled her own bottle of low-calorie salad dressing out of her bag, one friend was appalled, while the other applauded her. Obviously, it was the friend who applauded who became a reliable source of encouragement when it was needed. My patient knew that this friend wanted her to be at her best, and that made the friend a prime candidate for serving as a support 'system'.

It's that forgotten bite that can make the difference

Now let's suppose you're the parent of a child or teenager starting the Picture Perfect Weight Loss programme. Remember that your son or daughter must do this by and for himself or herself. Set the example. Be the role model. Serve as a support system. But don't interfere – no comments, no negative remarks. Let your children do their own thing; it's the only way they'll succeed. The best help you can give and the most powerful influence you can provide is to live the programme yourself.

STEP 3: START YOUR FOOD DIARY/PERSONAL JOURNAL

Somewhere in your notebook, write down your current weight. Call it your starting weight. Months from now, even weeks from now, you'll be thrilled with how far you've moved on from this number.

Now turn to the first blank page and start your Week 1 food diary. (The diary worksheet will change in the weeks to come.) The food diary is one of the most important tools of the Picture Perfect Weight Loss programme. It's the best way I know to understand your eating behaviour, and that understanding, in turn, is the best reason for changing your behaviour. For this reason, accuracy and attention to detail in keeping the food diary are absolutely essential.

Use the template shown on page 70 as a guide to creating your own food diary. Every time you eat anything – a meal or snack or 'bite' of anything at all – write it down in the diary immediately. This is important because we really do forget what we've eaten – and it's that forgotten bite that can make the difference, so 'catching up' on the diary later is never as effective as making your entries the minute you eat. And it's important also because keeping the diary faithfully is evidence of your commitment to the important mission you've undertaken – the mission of losing weight by changing your relationship with food.

BE SPECIFIC

Use your food diary to record the exact time and exactly what you ate. It's not enough to write 'soup and sandwich'. A cup of soup or a bowl? What flavour of soup? And what kind of sandwich? On what type of bread? Anything on it? With what drink?

> ### What mood were you in just before you ate?

Next, rank your desire to eat – at the time you ate the food – on a scale from 0 to 4, with 0 for no hunger at all and 4 for ravenous. Then fill in the entries that describe the circumstances in which you were eating. Were you alone or with others? If you were with other people, who were they? How many? What's your relationship with them – friend, spouse, colleague? Were you at home or out? If you were at home, make a note of which room you were in. If you were out, note if the location was a restaurant, a friend's house, or somewhere else. What mood were you in just before you ate? Were you bored, tense, happy, content, angry, tired, depressed? Write it down. Finally, jot down what else, if anything, you were doing at the time. Were you watching television, or perhaps reading in your favourite armchair? Whatever it was, write it down.

The importance of keeping the food diary – and doing so faithfully – cannot be overestimated. One patient of mine, himself a doctor, says that 'the diary confronts you with exactly what and when and what mental state you were in when you ate'. He claims that he

WEEK 1 FOOD DIARY

Date/Time	Food (Preparation, Serving Size)	Degree of Hunger (0–4)	People/Place	Mood	Activity

began losing weight as soon as he started keeping the food diary. And he stresses the 'keeping' part. 'In a stressful life, I tended to eat without thinking. I knew better, but knowing and doing are two different things,' he explained. 'Until I started keeping the food diary, that is. The diary was the incentive for constant and consistent awareness, and awareness was the incentive for consistently better choices.'

STEP 4: GET MOVING

We've talked about it throughout the book so far. We've discussed its importance for young people, older people and those in their middle years. Every health care professional you speak to, every new piece of research you hear about, every health column in every newspaper will confirm what you already know so well: exercise is good for you, and it's particularly good for you if you're trying to lose weight. Make up your mind that this week you will get moving – and you will continue to move for the rest of your life. And understand that 30 days from now, you are going to feel better and look better because you have begun to move.

For Week 1 of Picture Perfect Weight Loss, all I ask is that you start walking. This is an exercise you can do anytime, anywhere, in almost any weather. It doesn't require special equipment or mean you have to join a gym. All you need is a pair of sturdy, worn-in shoes, comfortable, loose-fitting shorts and a top. You don't even have to think of it as an exercise programme. Just go for a walk. Take the first steps to enjoying a healthy life. It really is that simple.

If you live in a city, walk a little further before getting on the bus or hailing a taxi. If you live in a flat, step out of the lift a few floors before your floor and take the stairs the rest of the way up. Head for the nearest park: walk across it or around it – or both.

If you live in a house with stairs, walk up and down them a few times in succession. Stride back and forth across your garden. Take a walk down the street; explore your neighbourhood. Walk to the newsagents to buy that item you forgot to get yesterday . . . or to the library to return a book . . . or to a neighbour's house just to say 'hello'.

Walk briskly. Swing your arms. Move those legs. Breathe deeply. You don't have to run, or get out of breath, or sweat. All you have to do is *move*. And keep moving.

As with food awareness, exercise awareness will eventually become second nature to you, and exercise itself will become a part of everything you do. It won't be 'exercise' anymore; it will be lifestyle physical activity – and it starts right now in Week 1.

STEP 5: DISCOVER NEW CHOICES FOR BREAKFAST

'Breakfast is the most important meal of the day.' That's the standard cliché, and people sometimes feel guilty if they don't sit down to a proper meal for breakfast, or if their morning appetite is sated with only a cup of coffee or a mug of tea. In my view, that guilt is unfounded. If you're not hungry, you don't

> ## Walk briskly. Swing your arms. Move those legs

really need to have breakfast at all. Except for children, that is. They really do benefit from a nutritious morning meal. Study after study shows that kids who eat a nourishing breakfast do better at school and develop more healthily than children who do not have breakfast.

Don't make the mistake of denying yourself breakfast to 'save' calories, though. The denial will only come back to haunt you during the

Soya products are so good for us in so many ways

day. Biology will take over and prompt you to eat more — and to eat higher-calorie foods. As always, deprivation backfires. Skip breakfast if you're not hungry, but not because you think fasting in the morning will help you lose weight. It won't.

WHAT'S NEW?

Your goal for Week 1 should be to try something new for breakfast. In fact, I'm going to recommend that three of the week's seven breakfasts include foods you've never eaten before. Been eating the same cereal for the past 20 years? Find something new this week. Always eaten cheese omelettes every other day? This is the week to discover an alternative. Adding new tastes to your palate is a boon to your state of mind as well. As psychotherapist Susan Amato puts it, it's a 'reminder that you're adding good things to your life — and to your kitchen — not subtracting'.

NUTRITION TO START YOUR DAY OFF THE RIGHT WAY

I want to offer two main guidelines for thinking in a fresh way about your first meal of the day. Both will give you an excellent start in obtaining the nutrition you need.

Include fruit (and/or vegetables) in your breakfast. Adding fruit to your breakfast choices is a great way to start — a banana in your cereal, melon with berries, an apple with

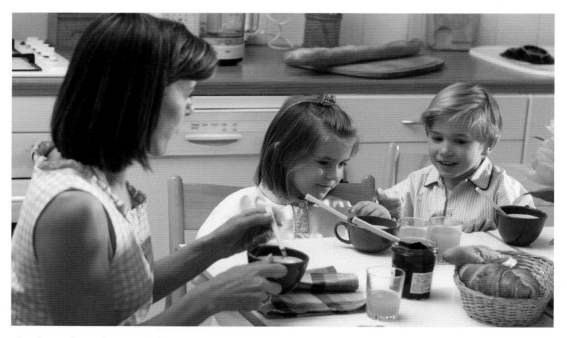

The benefits of breakfast
Studies have shown that children who eat breakfast are healthier, happier and even perform better academically than those who miss out on a morning meal.

NOTES ON OATS

Oats are high in protein, rich in soluble fibre and an excellent source of thiamin, or vitamin B1. The particular kind of fibre they contain is called beta glucan, and it is particularly effective in lowering the 'bad' LDL cholesterol that can endanger coronary arteries. Oat fibre may also lower high blood pressure and help control blood sugar. As a plant food, oats contain disease-fighting phytochemicals that may reduce heart disease risk, relax blood vessels and maintain bloodflow.

Get your oats in any form of oatmeal, fibre-rich oat bran, and a number of breakfast cereals and breads. Make sure the label says 'wholegrain oats', and look for products with at least two grams of fibre per serving.

a bagel. You can also use breakfast to get a head start on the day's vegetable intake by choosing a vegetable omelette, or maybe eggs Florentine (with spinach).

Introduce soya into your life. Soya products are so good for us in so many ways, and breakfast is a great way to experiment. Try soya milk with cereal, or tuck into a couple of vegetarian sausages.

SOME BREAKFAST IDEAS

Now, let's put it all together in some breakfast suggestions. Remember: these ideas are just a starting point. Expand your breakfast repertoire with the food demonstrations pictured in this chapter. But as you become increasingly aware of what you eat, let your own imagination and newly expanding palate guide you to more breakfast choices.

■ **Cereal for breakfast** Go for a low-calorie, wholegrain or high-fibre cereal. Accompany it with low-fat soya milk or skimmed milk. Finally, add fresh and/or dried fruit to the bowl.

■ **Coffee and . . .** If your idea of a good breakfast is a piece of toast or a roll with coffee, make it light toast or a wholegrain roll. Spread jam on it. And by all means, add a piece of fruit or even a plate of fruit. Remember: fibre is your friend!

■ **For kids** Many of the breakfast foods geared towards children make great Picture Perfect Weight Loss breakfasts. A great number are low-calorie and wholegrain, so all you need to do is introduce soya milk or skimmed milk to give your child a weight-loss boost.

All of the suggestions I've listed also work for children, of course. These ideas are a great way to push kids' palates towards a more healthy, nutritious, low-calorie breakfast habit.

YOUR WEEK 1 GOALS

◆ Weigh yourself – and write down your starting weight.

◆ Start your food diary. Make it a personal journal as well.

◆ Commit to 10 minutes of exercise per day. Get moving.

◆ Begin to change your eating habits by making every breakfast you eat a Picture Perfect Weight Loss breakfast.

◆ Eat a food you've never tried before for three of the week's seven breakfasts.

EAT FRUIT, DON'T DRINK IT

Check out the high calorie count of the juice on the left. Instead, you can have your fruit and drink it too – without wasting calories. It's proof that you're better off drinking a low-calorie, reduced-sugar drink and taking in the rich nutrients and fibre in the real thing.

If you absolutely cannot stand the idea of eating delicious, refreshing, vitamin-packed fruit, then consider purchasing a juicer or smoothie maker. Simply throw in fresh fruit, a dash of low-calorie, reduced sugar drink, and then whizz up an instant serving of fruity goodness.

'Fruit contains plenty of fibre, which is good both for your health and for giving you that "full" feeling.'

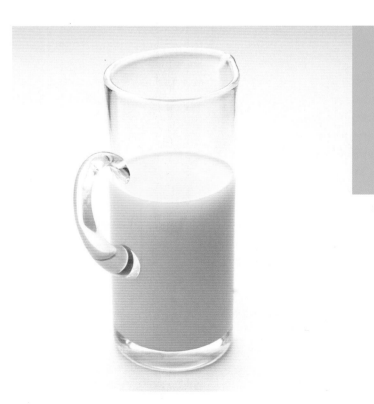

orange juice (1 litre)

425 calories

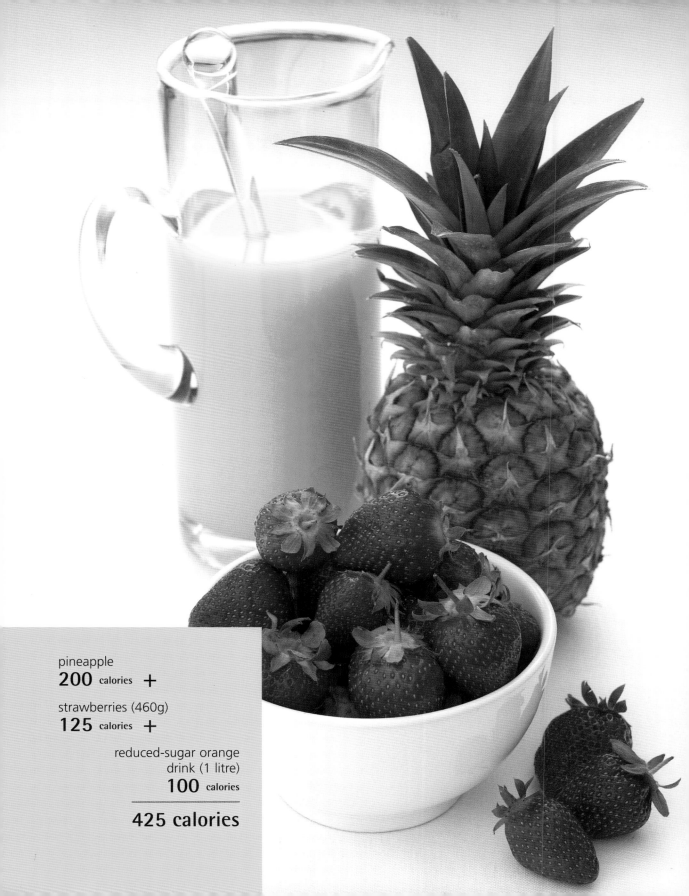

pineapple
200 calories **+**

strawberries (460g)
125 calories **+**

reduced-sugar orange
drink (1 litre)
100 calories

425 calories

CEREAL KILLER

Beware the cereal with the oh-so-healthy-sounding name. It may be crunchy and full of taste, but it can also mean a high-calorie start to the day. For the same bowl of oat, honey and raisin cereal on the left,

'Sweet oat cereals often taste like cookies – so it's no wonder that they're full of calories.'

you can enjoy all four bowls of cereal on the right – with strawberries – and polish them off with a cafetiere of filter coffee. One other word of caution about these supposedly healthy kinds of cereal: they're all too easy to snack on right out of the box – at any time of the day – making them a real calorie culprit.

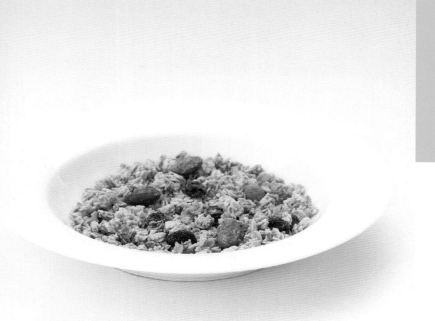

oat, honey and raisin
cereal (80g)

450 calories

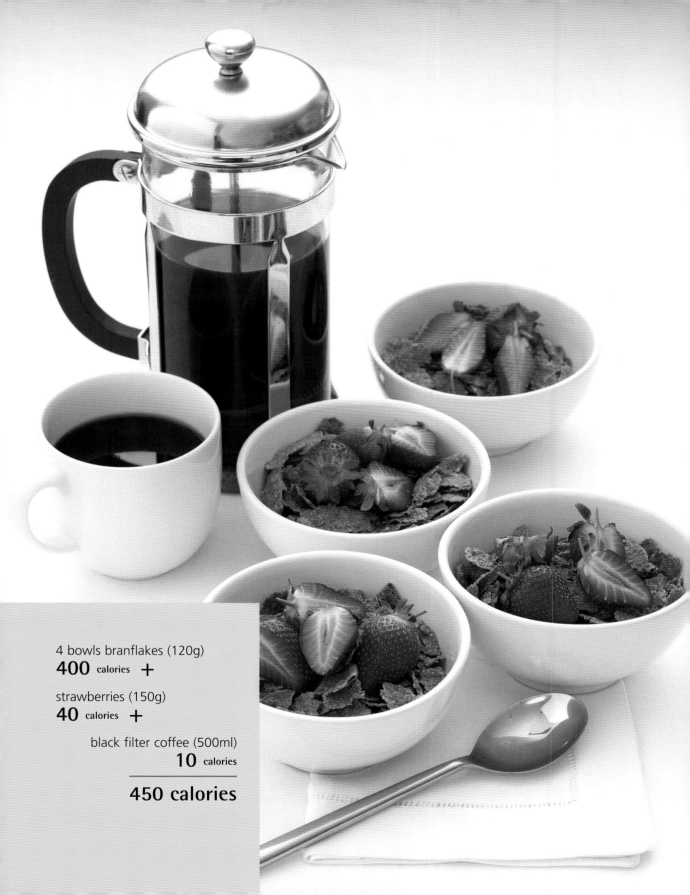

4 bowls branflakes (120g)
400 calories **+**

strawberries (150g)
40 calories **+**

black filter coffee (500ml)
10 calories
___

450 calories

BERRY NICE INDEED

In a hurry? How much longer does it take to pop a couple of waffles in the toaster than to do the same with fruit pockets? The answer? It takes no more time. And why waste calories eating fruit pockets just to save a few seconds? Save the calories instead – and enjoy the taste and good nutrition of waffles with a generous serving of fresh mixed berries and a tablespoon of syrup.

'As well as vitamin C, many types of berry contain ellagic acid, which may help to fight cancer.'

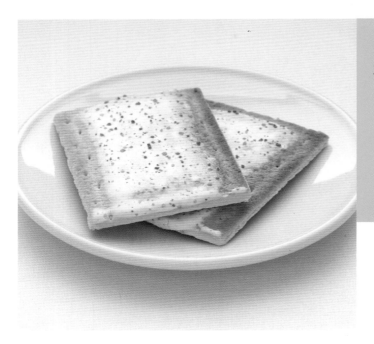

2 fruit pockets

470 calories

VS

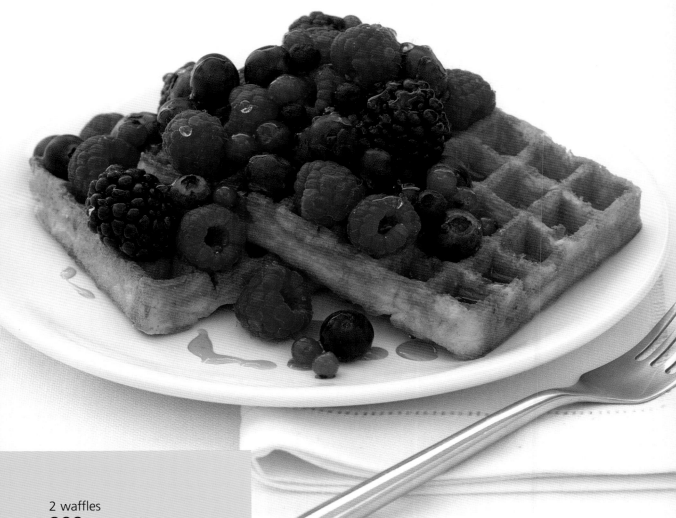

2 waffles
300 calories **+**

mixed berries (35g)
10 calories **+**

syrup (1 tbsp)
60 calories
_____

370 calories

'This serving of fruit and waffles will satisfy anyone's craving for something sweet at breakfast.'

RAISE A TOAST

For the weight-conscious, light bread can serve an important function – and it's a lot tastier than many people think. It would take seven slices of light-bread toast, each spread with reduced-sugar jam, to equal just one pain au chocolat. What's more, the pain au chocolat contains 'bad', saturated fat, while the light bread is a good source of fibre.

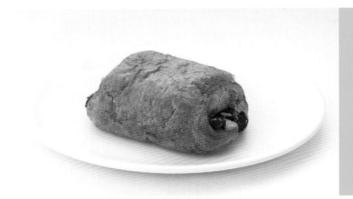

pain au chocolate
___
410 calories

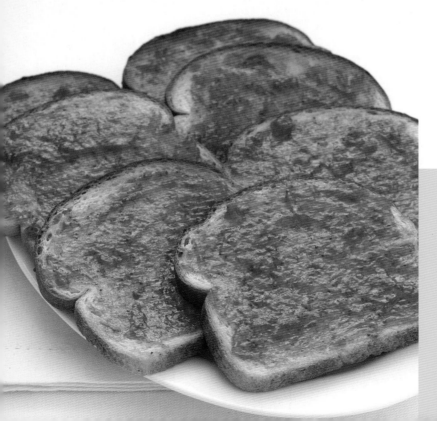

7 slices of light toast
315 calories **+**

reduced-sugar jam (7 tbsp)
95 calories
___
410 calories

BANANAS FOR BAGELS

Bagels are a very popular food; we eat them for breakfast, we eat them for lunch – they're good to eat anytime. But, alas, the bagel is high in refined carbohydrates and offers no nutritional benefit. If it's nutritional benefit you're after, try a banana. They're full of fibre, and when it comes to calories, three bananas are equal to one medium-sized bagel.

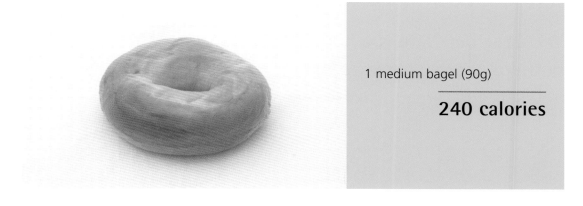

1 medium bagel (90g)

240 calories

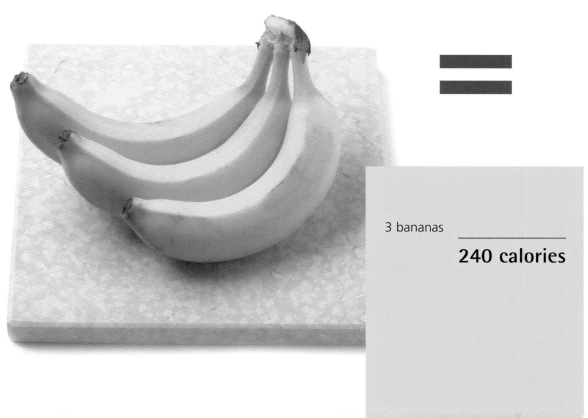

3 bananas

240 calories

A CONTINENTAL CLASSIC

A cheese omelette is quick and easy to prepare, but it's lacking in different flavours, textures and nutrients – plus it's groaning under the weight of the calories it contains. Why not get your protein from a boiled egg and a small piece of cheese (or fish or soya products), fibre from the bread, and the goodness of fresh salad from the tomatoes and cucumber? And there you have it: lots of flavours, a variety of textures, and a whole host of nutrients.

'A cheese omelette is a high-calorie and low-nutrient choice compared with a meal of a boiled egg, bread, cheese and salad.'

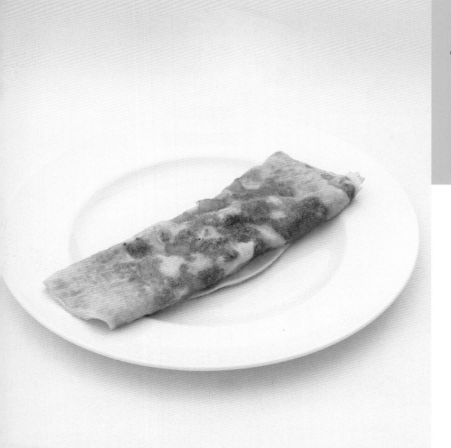

cheese omelette (100g)

500 calories

VS

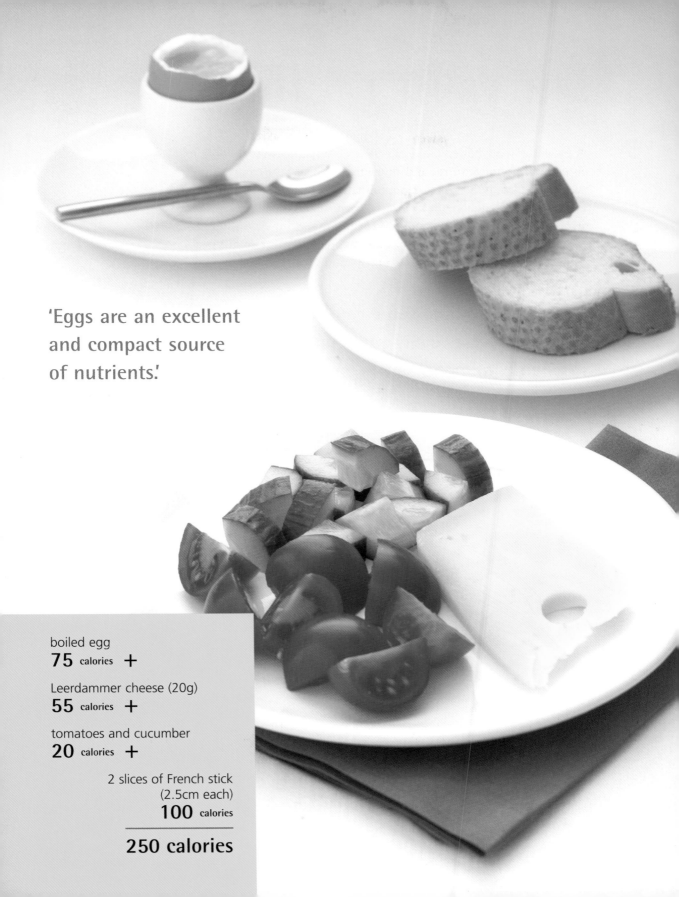

'Eggs are an excellent
and compact source
of nutrients.'

boiled egg
75 calories **+**

Leerdammer cheese (20g)
55 calories **+**

tomatoes and cucumber
20 calories **+**

2 slices of French stick
(2.5cm each)
100 calories

---

250 calories

THE FRUIT FACTOR

A croissant with butter looks harmless enough, doesn't it? Not the most calorific food on the planet, is it? This may be so, but it's only when you look at the croissant opposite the banana and mixed berries, the slice of watermelon, the serving of yoghurt and the wholemeal roll with jam that you realise what you're missing out on. And if you eat the food on the right for breakfast, think how much more full you'll feel – right up till lunchtime – than if you opt for the croissant.

'More food for the same calories is always a bargain – especially when you also get more nourishment.'

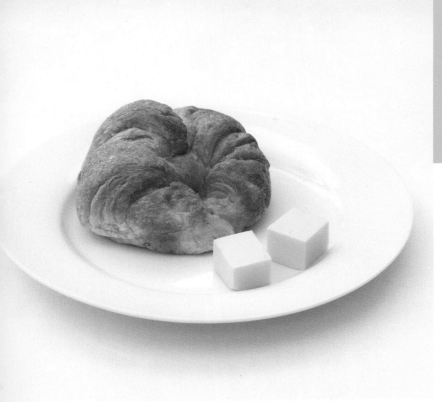

1 croissant (67g)
250 calories **+**

2 cubes of butter (48g)
180 calories

_____

430 calories

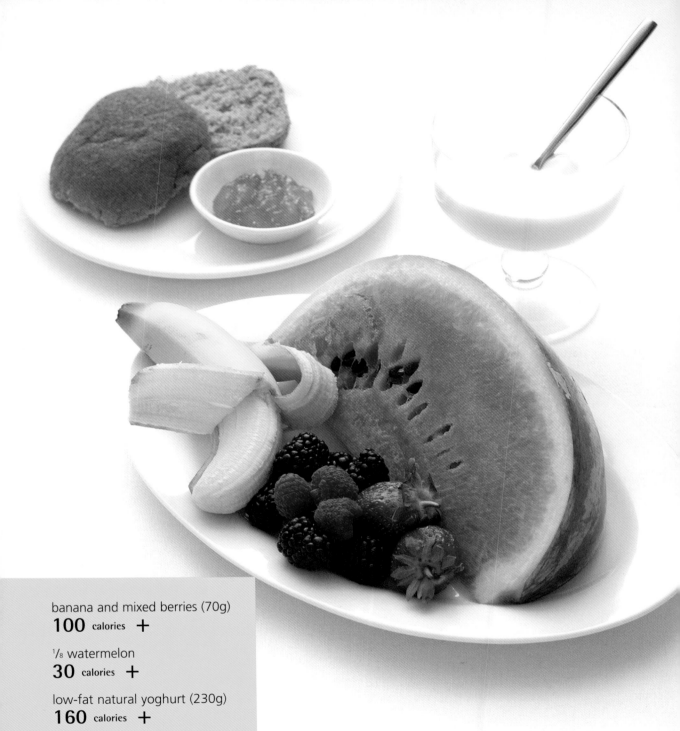

banana and mixed berries (70g)
100 calories **+**

¹⁄₈ watermelon
30 calories **+**

low-fat natural yoghurt (230g)
160 calories **+**

wholemeal roll (40g)
100 calories **+**

reduced-sugar jam (3 tbsp)
40 calories

───────────────

430 calories

'Adding fruit to your breakfast is a great way to start the day – choose any fruit you like.'

CHAPTER 5: WEEK 2 – A NEW VIEW OF LUNCH AND SNACKS

YOUR WEEK 2 AGENDA

By the end of Week 2, you will have:
◆ Figured out your emotional connection with food.
◆ Begun to make physical activity an integral part of your lifestyle.
◆ Tried some new lunch ideas – including soya.
◆ Discovered a new way to snack.
◆ Lost more weight.

Whether you're at work, at home or at a five-star restaurant . . . whether you're grabbing something on the run or cooking for yourself or waiting in the canteen queue, lunch can and *should* be a tasty, satisfying, healthy meal that is also low in calories. In fact, lunch is a great time to put the principles of Picture Perfect Weight Loss to work.

FROM LUNCHTIME TO SNACK TIME: SEVEN STEPS TO KEEP THE MOMENTUM GOING

The issue may be more than just wondering 'what's for lunch?'. After all, you're in Week 2 of a four-week programme to change your life, change your relationship with food, and change the way you look and feel.

If this were a diet, and you had survived a week of it, you would probably be feeling pretty deprived. But Picture Perfect Weight Loss isn't about taking foods away from you; it's about adding to your food choices. You're not on a diet: you're on a journey, and you're about to move into stage two of the journey.

You need a new goal to get the energy going again

Each stage – each of the four weeks of the Picture Perfect Weight Loss 30 Day Plan – teaches you something new.

Last week, I offered five steps to getting started on your commitment to change – and to a whole new view of breakfast. This week offers a seven-step plan to new ideas about lunch and snacks – and to ways of keeping the momentum of change going.

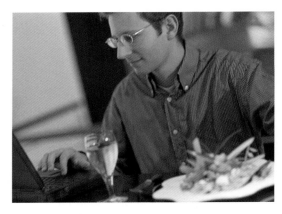

Make a date for lunch
Wherever you find yourself come lunchtime, the Picture Perfect Weight Loss programme allows you always to eat a delicious and nutritious meal.

STEP 1: WHAT ARE YOU REALLY FEELING?

Week 1 was the start of a fundamental change in your life – a novelty – and you were revved up. You were curious and enthusiastic. You lost weight – you were a success. But this is Week 2. The high of the first week is not as great. Why? And more importantly, what should you do next? You need a new goal to get the energy going again – the kind of energy generated by positive change.

Part of the reason for the slump you may be experiencing can be found in the Week 1 food diary you kept. Take a look at it now, paying particular attention to the descriptive points: degree of hunger, people you were with, place, mood, activity. Can you find an emotional pattern in these measures? Dr Adele Fink, the psychologist we met earlier, recommends thinking about your emotional pattern in terms of four categories of feeling: sad, mad, bad and glad. Does your pattern show that you tended to eat higher-calorie foods when you felt sad – lonely, lost, bored, unhappy with yourself, or just plain depressed? Did you eat when you were angry, when sheer rage made you uncomfortable? Did you eat out of anxiety or fear or when feeling the bad effects of stress? Did you eat to celebrate something – or because you just felt glad? In other words, what were the feelings that 'governed' your eating – that influenced your need to eat, the choices you made, the foods that satisfied you?

> ### Instead of 'eating' feelings, you'll learn to feel them

Once you understand how you use food to disconnect from your real feelings, you can begin in Week 2 to get in touch with them. Instead of 'eating' those feelings, you'll learn to feel them – and return food to its real purpose in your life: nutrition and enjoyment.

STEP 2: BREAK THE CYCLE

You have also previously met Susan Amato, the psychotherapist who works with me in my New York office. As Susan says: 'Change is the essence of the entire Picture Perfect Weight Loss programme, and to keep the ball rolling, you have to keep changing.' In Week 2, Susan suggests you break the cycle of the behaviour that has been giving you the most difficulty. She cites the case of one patient who found

FIGHT CANCER WITH EXERCISE

You know that exercise promotes heart health and burns calories. Now an exercise research facility has demonstrated that regular aerobic exercise – like a brisk walk, vigorous housework and even gardening – may also fight cancer. One study followed 20,000 men for more than 10 years and found that lower heart and lung fitness correlated with double the risk of death from cancer. Another study looked at lung cancer in 25,000 men and found that the unfit had almost four times the risk faced by fitter men. The reason? Researchers suggest that since carcinogens accumulate in fat cells, exercise that lowers body-fat stores can protect against cancer. So don't just sit there – get up and exercise!

she nibbled high-calorie snacks constantly while preparing the family dinner in the evening. Susan's suggestion? Do the dinner prep work in the morning. That change alone focused the patient's mind and made her conscious of what she put in her mouth.

The mere act of change – the breaking of the cycle – can produce a ripple effect of benefits. It takes your focus off whatever it is that you're finding difficult and puts the focus

> ## This is your life, your weight and your programme

on your goal. Since Picture Perfect Weight Loss is all about change – changing your relationship with food and changing your eating habits – that's all the better. So breaking the cycle is an important step in keeping the momentum going.

STEP 3: FIND YOUR VOICE

In Week 1, we talked about 'honouring thyself' – taking time *for* yourself and taking care *of* yourself. In Week 2, it's time to take it a step further, find your voice and assert yourself. Here are three rules for finding your voice:

■ **Any interest shown by your family and friends in the changes you're making for Picture Perfect Weight Loss can be only in the form of support.** That means no criticism. It also means none of the kind of 'encouragement' that leads to irritation, as in: 'Are you sure you want to eat that slice of cheesecake?' As you well know, such queries, innocent though they may be, are not helpful. Speak up, and make it clear that this is *your* life, *your* weight and *your* programme, and that you'll accept unconditional support – or silence. And the same goes for you vis-à-vis your children: it's *their* lives, *their* weight and *their* programme – so give them your unconditional support, not negativity.

■ **Set clear boundaries.** Stop being a doormat. Remember the woman on the exercise bike in the previous chapter who never found time for herself? It's essential to separate the areas of your life that belong to you from those areas into which you will accept or invite others. Only by setting these boundaries can you keep safe the effort you're making now to lose weight once and for all.

■ **Remember that what the bathroom scales tell you is not the barometer of success.** Scales measure only your weight

THE GYM IN YOUR GARDEN

Weeding, digging, pruning, raking and mowing. Spend time working in your garden, and you can give yourself a vigorous all-around exercise workout. Scientists confirm that the tasks of gardening can strengthen your heart and lungs, enhance flexibility and serve as resistance exercises that build muscle strength. Two tips to think about as you work:

first, bend from your knees, not your back. Second, alternate movements. Don't spend all day squatting down to weed. Instead, do a little weeding, then stand up and switch to pruning, then switch to shovelling, then switch again to weeding, and so on. Keep these different movements going, otherwise you run the risk of repetitive motion injuries.

loss. The real measure of success is your willingness to undertake the journey in the first place.

STEP 4: TIME TO WRITE YOUR WEEK 2 FOOD DIARY

Your Week 1 food diary was meant to serve as the boost that helped jump-start you towards Picture Perfect Weight Loss. The purpose of the Week 2 food diary is to keep your awareness level high as you continue to transform your eating habits and incorporate Picture Perfect Weight Loss into your life. You'll find the Week 2 diary on page 90.

The most important part of the Week 2 food diary is what you'll learn when you review it at the end of the week. Why at the end of the week? Because you can always justify a high-calorie or 'bad' food choice at the time you decide to eat it. But the end-of-the-week review gives you a real grasp of the frequency of your inappropriate choices and the justification you create for eating them – and can show you how to change the behaviour that led to those particular choices.

STEP 5: LIFESTYLE EXERCISE

Lifestyle exercise is the exercise you do around the house or as part of daily activities such as going to the shops or doing your job. For Week 2 of the Picture Perfect Weight Loss 30 Day Plan, I want you to start thinking about these physical activities, to become aware of them, and to do them with care and deliberation.

Lifestyle exercise embraces the three components of physical activity that are so essential to a lifetime of fitness: aerobic exercise, strength training and flexibility. Why are all three essential? Aerobic exercise – walking, cycling, dancing, climbing stairs – works your heart, lungs and circulatory system while also building your endurance.

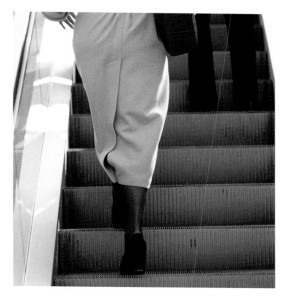

Fit for life
Lifestyle exercise is something that you don't even have to incorporate into your life: you do it *every* day, from walking to cleaning to climbing the stairs.

Strength training – lifting weights or carrying the shopping – builds muscle tissue, and built-up muscles are best at burning calories. What's more, this kind of weight-bearing exercise, as

The more lifestyle exercise you do, the more you can do

it is also called, counteracts the loss of muscle mass and the potential development of osteoporosis that are both signs of ageing. So do flexibility activities – anything from a weekly yoga session to pulling weeds or hanging pictures or making the bed. Such stretching is the key to preventing injury, improving balance and co-ordination, and keeping you supple as you grow older.

For all these reasons, making lifestyle exercise as automatic as choosing low-calorie foods is essential to Picture Perfect Weight Loss. And as with any physical activity, the more lifestyle exercise you do, the more you *can* do. For Week 2 of the 30 Day Plan, therefore, I'm setting you two exercise assignments.

■ **Keep moving.** Last week, you started walking. This week, make sure you do a brisk walk of at least 10 minutes every day.

■ **Make physical activity part of your lifestyle.** Whenever and wherever there's an opportunity to burn calories, seize it: be aware that you're doing a physical activity, and make it count.

STEP 6: WHAT'S FOR LUNCH?

It's the middle of the day, and you're hungry. You've been at work, or you've tidied the house, or you've been on the move, and you're ready to eat something – especially if you didn't bother with breakfast this morning.

Where lunch is concerned, branch out. That's your basic assignment for this week: at least four days out of the seven, eat something for lunch you've never had before – either because you didn't know about it, or because you simply wouldn't have considered it. Make one of your four 'new' lunches a soya-product lunch – maybe a veggie burger, or tofu and vegetable kebabs, for example.

Apart from that one requirement, however, your new lunches are up to you. Here are some guidelines that all the Picture Perfect Weight Loss 'graduates' have found useful.

■ **Think soup and a salad.** Soup and a salad is the lunch of choice for Picture Perfect Weight Loss. The combination is a high-fibre meal that satisfies the appetite and fills the stomach, nourishes the body and keeps the calorie count down.

WEEK 2 FOOD DIARY

Date/Time	Food (Preparation, Serving Size)	Comments

When I talk about soup, I mean a hearty concoction with plenty of body. If your choice contains pulses and vegetables, you're getting an added bonus in fibre, nutrition and satisfaction. A good soup is a meal in itself; if it's not, add a salad.

■ **Load your salads with vegetables.** But go easy on the high-calorie garnishes. And by vegetables, I mean all vegetables: raw, pickled,

> A good soup is a meal in itself; if it's not, add a salad

marinated . . . lettuces, carrots, red and yellow peppers, beetroot, mushrooms . . . artichoke hearts and coleslaw. Make your salad as varied in colour, texture and ingredients as possible.

■ **Be sure to keep dressings low in calories.** A clear oil-and-vinegar dressing is not necessarily lower in calories than the creamy-looking choice at the salad bar. If you do use oil and vinegar, go easy on the oil; at 120 calories per tablespoon, it can all soon add up. Also beware of classic vinaigrette at 70 to 100 calories per tablespoon. If you're eating out for lunch, ask for a light dressing or oil and vinegar on the side.

■ **Reinvent the sandwich.** Instead of your usual sandwich – filled with as much cheese and ham as possible, maybe? – satisfy your cravings for fillings with just a taste, fill up on salads and try using light bread instead of high-calorie slices.

■ **Know that not every burger is a beef burger.** A beef burger is a high-calorie item, and it can also be expensive in terms of your health – especially heart health. So what are the alternatives? There are *loads* of alternatives. Try a turkey burger, a tuna sandwich, a portobello mushroom sandwich or a vegetarian burger.

STEP 7: THE SNACK BETWEEN MEALS

It's 3pm and you're hungry again – even though you had lunch a couple of hours ago. You need to eat, but how can you satisfy the craving and still keep the number of calories you consume low?

Probably your best bet is fruit. Fruit contains plenty of fibre, which is good both for your health and for giving you that 'full' feeling. But if fruit doesn't satisfy your sweet tooth, I recommend boiled sweets or low-calorie frozen desserts. The calorie counts are fine for those watching their weight: a lollipop weighs in at 50 to 60 calories, while an ice pop contains only 30 to 40 calories.

If something salty is more to your liking, think about breadsticks. These have long been part of the healthy Mediterranean diet. The average breadstick contains fewer than 30 calories and is ideal for snacking.

YOUR WEEK 2 GOALS

◆ Review your Week 1 food diary. What does it say about your feelings associated with eating?

◆ Break the cycle of an unhealthy habit – then keep the momentum going.

◆ Find your voice: assert your needs.

◆ Start your Week 2 food diary.

◆ Walk briskly for at least 10 minutes every day, and start making physical activity an integral part of your lifestyle.

◆ For four days out of the seven, have something brand new for lunch. Include a soup-and-salad combination and a soya product.

◆ Change your snack habits to fruits, boiled sweets or low-calorie frozen desserts.

MAGIC MUSHROOM

Portobello mushrooms – the huge Italian fungi – are a rich-tasting alternative to meat. On a seeded roll, the grilled Portobello mushroom and a dollop of Dijon mustard undercuts the calorie count of a roast beef sandwich by more than two-thirds. Replace a high-fat choice with a nutritious, low-fat option like this just once a day, and you're bound to experience weight loss.

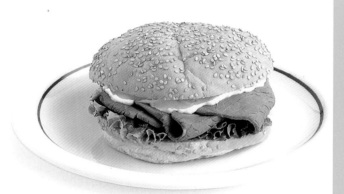

roast beef slices (75g)
280 calories **+**

seeded roll
180 calories **+**

mayonnaise (2 tbsp)
220 calories

_____

680 calories

VS

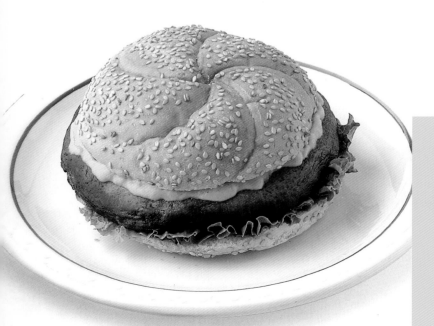

large Portobello mushroom
20 calories **+**

seeded roll
180 calories **+**

Dijon mustard (1 tbsp)
20 calories

_____

220 calories

SIZE MATTERS

You're in a hurry. You need to grab something to eat that you can prepare and polish off in minutes. Check out the tiny cube of cheese below. It requires no preparation and you'll have finished it before you know it – and still be hungry. Another option is a bowl full of nutritious soup – with a slice of French stick. Same calorie count, lots more food and a healthier way to eat when time is tight.

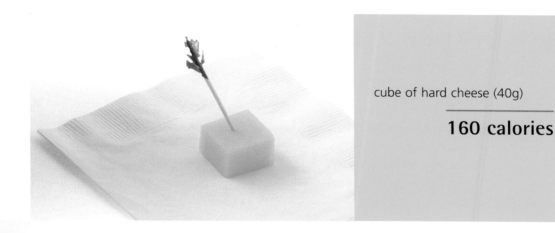

cube of hard cheese (40g)
_____

160 calories

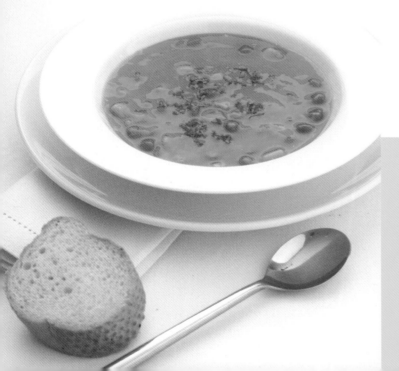

vegetable soup (220ml)
110 calories **+**

slice of French stick (2.5cm)
50 calories
_____

160 calories

FANTASTIC FRITTATA

Croque Monsieur is the classic French toasted ham and cheese sandwich of café society fame. It conjures up visions of crowded, atmospheric Parisian pavement cafés on hot, sunny days – the waft of food in the air making you hungry. Never mind the vision though: the reality is that the ham and cheese in Croque Monsieur come at a high calorific price. For the same number of calories, why not enjoy a larger

'We all love cheese, and we all know that it's high in fat – the kind of saturated fat we should all try to limit.'

meal, starting with a delicious bowl of onion soup before moving onto a generous slice of frittata and a side salad with low-fat dressing. As if that wasn't incentive enough, you can also accompany your meal with a glass of white wine. *Bon appetit!*

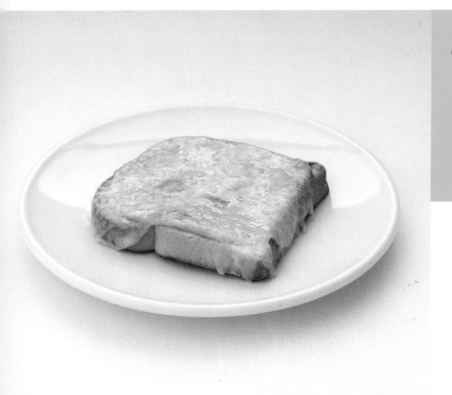

Croque Monsieur

460 calories

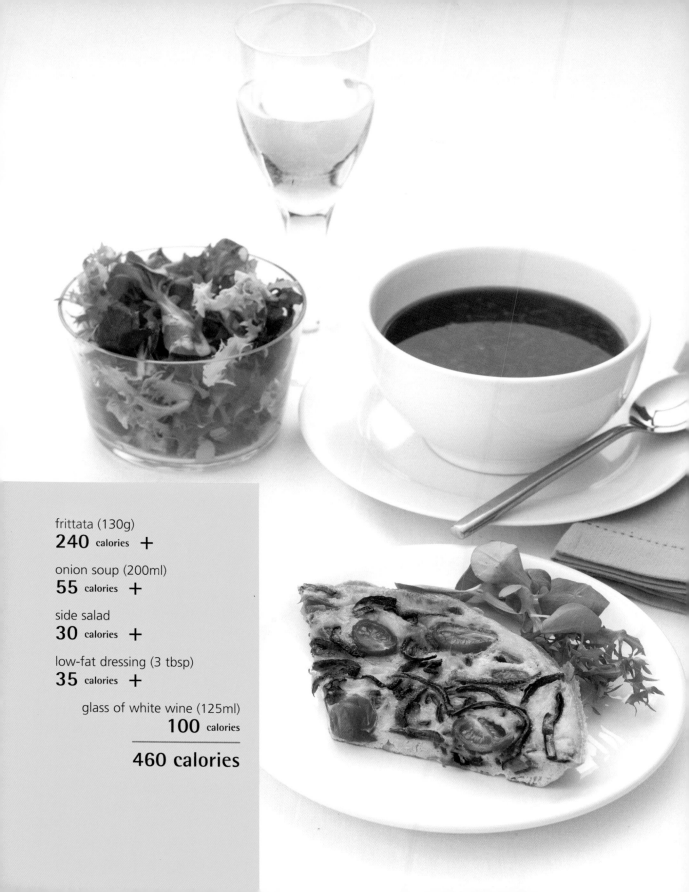

frittata (130g)
240 calories **+**

onion soup (200ml)
55 calories **+**

side salad
30 calories **+**

low-fat dressing (3 tbsp)
35 calories **+**

glass of white wine (125ml)
100 calories
_____

460 calories

IT'S A WRAP

Wraps have become an extremely popular choice for lunches and snacks, but some can be high in calories despite their modest size. The vegetable wrap beats the Brie wrap by a mile in calorie count and healthiness, making it a great way to take in vegetables, and the serving of hummus gives it a little added zing for minimal calories.

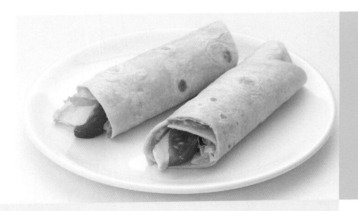

Brie tortilla wrap (55g)
_____

740 calories

VS

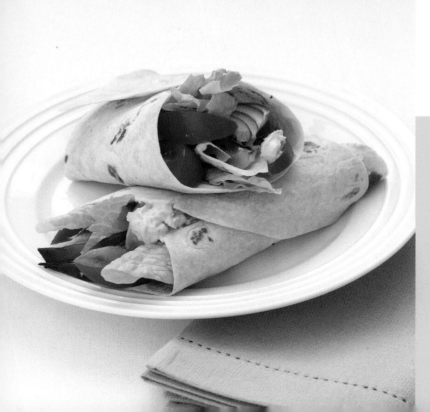

tortilla wrap (55g)
170 calories **+**

grilled mixed peppers (20g)
20 calories **+**

grilled red onion (30g)
10 calories **+**

tomato and lettuce
20 calories **+**

hummus (25g)
50 calories
_____

270 calories

SOYA SORCERY

So, you've always had a quarter-pounder cheeseburger with bacon for lunch? Well, you're just throwing calories away. Lose two-thirds of the calories simply by changing your choice of burger. For a huge health bonus, choose soya every time: it's full of protein, it contains many important nutrients, and it can even help prevent many cancers.

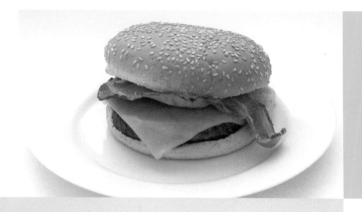

quarter-pounder cheeseburger
with bacon

_____

660 calories

VS

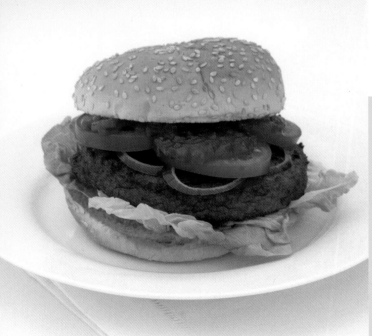

veggie burger:
soya burger (60g)
80 calories **+**

bun (50g)
120 calories **+**

lettuce, tomato,
onion and relish
20 calories

_____

220 calories

A SAUSAGE SENSATION

Soya products are gradually becoming part of everyday life, and it's no surprise: they're a wonder food. As well as being delicious, the soya used in the veggie sausages below is a healthy, low-calorie alternative to the traditional meat sausage. What's more, as a protein source, soya is comparable to meat and eggs. And with less than two-thirds of the calories of meat sausages, soya sausages win every time.

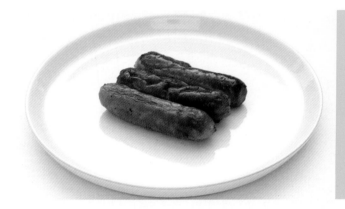

3 meat sausages
_____
550 calories

VS

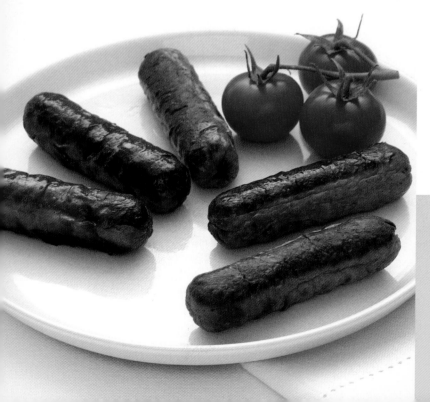

5 veggie sausages
270 calories **+**

tomatoes (100g)
20 calories
_____
290 calories

A CHOICE OF CHILLI

Soya has been cultivated for at least 5000 years, and there are 2500 varieties of soya under cultivation. It comes in many forms – as tofu, roasted soya nuts, miso and soya milk. Possibly one of the best uses of soya, though, is as a tasty, healthy, low-calorie substitute for minced beef in chilli, as shown here. You probably won't be able to taste the difference between the two, and you'll save yourself 330 calories.

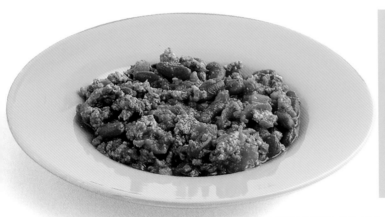

meat chilli (500g)

610 calories

VS

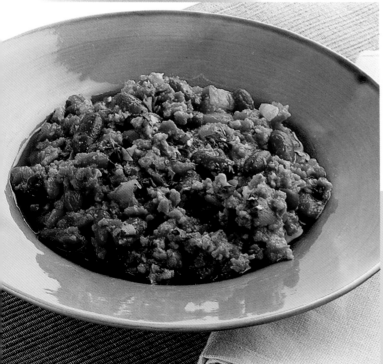

veggie chilli (500g)

280 calories

POTATO PERFECTION

Where the 'side dish' is concerned, think potatoes. In fact, for the weight-conscious, the potato is a powerful secret weapon – when it isn't chipped. Baked white and sweet potatoes are satisfying and nutritious, and lend themselves to a range of culinary possibilities. The

'Fries are high in fat. In fact, you'll consume more calories from the frying fat than from the potato.'

ones shown on the right offer just an idea of what can be done with different toppings and condiments. For health, nutrition and calorie count, any of these dishes is a far better bet than the French fries pictured below, which are calorifically expensive and not all that filling.

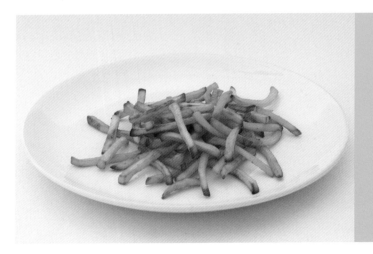

large fries (180g)

660 calories

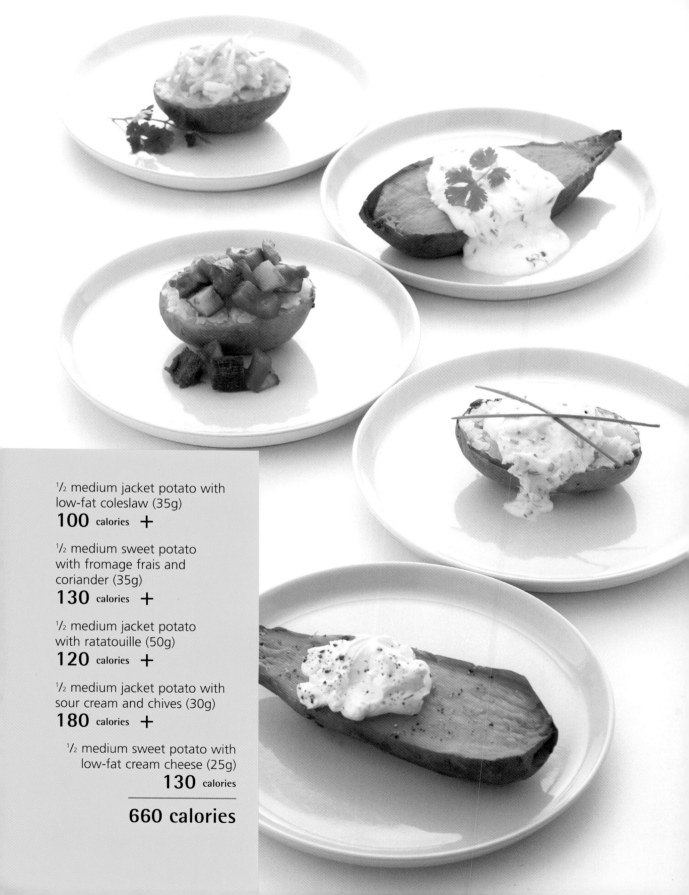

¹/₂ medium jacket potato with low-fat coleslaw (35g)
100 calories **+**

¹/₂ medium sweet potato with fromage frais and coriander (35g)
130 calories **+**

¹/₂ medium jacket potato with ratatouille (50g)
120 calories **+**

¹/₂ medium jacket potato with sour cream and chives (30g)
180 calories **+**

¹/₂ medium sweet potato with low-fat cream cheese (25g)
130 calories

660 calories

BREADSTICK BENEFITS

Crisps . . . you just *know* that they're not good for people who are watching their weight. So don't eat them. Instead of wolfing down a bag of the high-calorie critters – laden with fat – you're much better off munching on a few breadsticks, which are delicious and low in calories. Breadsticks are ideal for snacking on when you're starving and waiting for your dinner to cook.

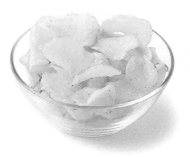

plain crisps (60g)

320 calories

=

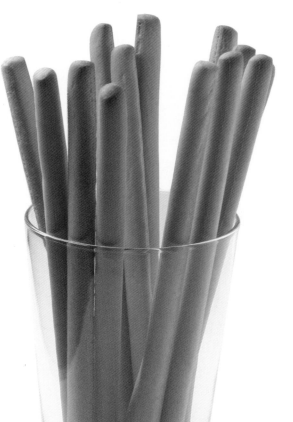

breadsticks (80g)

320 calories

A PASSION FOR POPCORN

Tropical fruit-and-nut mixes are deceptive. They're deceptive because people generally believe that they make a healthy snack. And they do – to a degree. But these kinds of mixes are also chock-full of calories. When you really want to nibble on something healthy, popcorn is a great choice. Just look at the demonstration: *see* how much more food you can eat for the same number of calories.

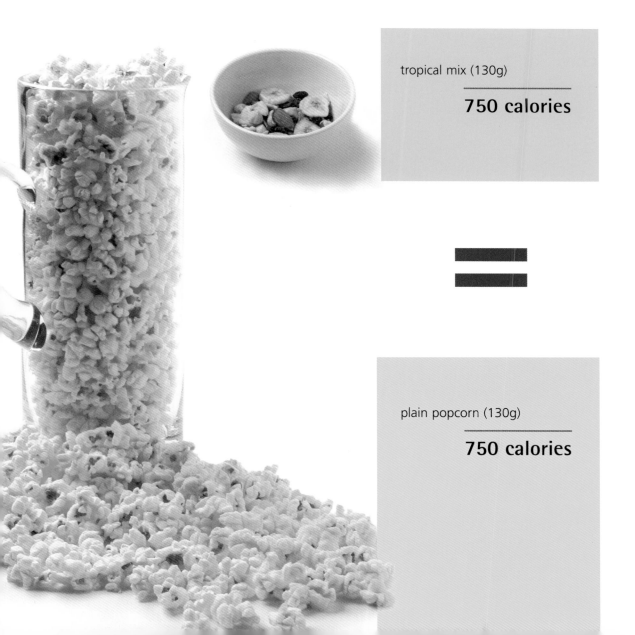

tropical mix (130g)
_____
750 calories

plain popcorn (130g)
_____
750 calories

NOT SO SMOOTH

Some advice to the weight-conscious: eat your calories, don't drink them. Eating real fruit beats a fruit drink every time. Except, that is, if you make a smoothie using only fruit and real fruit juice. The smoothie below has been made using ice cream and honey, which has bumped the calories right up. Look on the right at all the food and drink you can consume for 140 calories less.

'If it's a "hit" of sweetness you crave, go for sorbet, which offers great taste and is low in calories.'

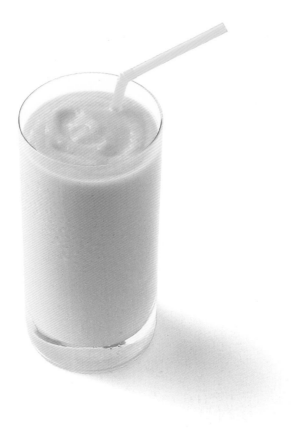

strawberry and banana
ice-cream smoothie (300ml)

400 calories

VS

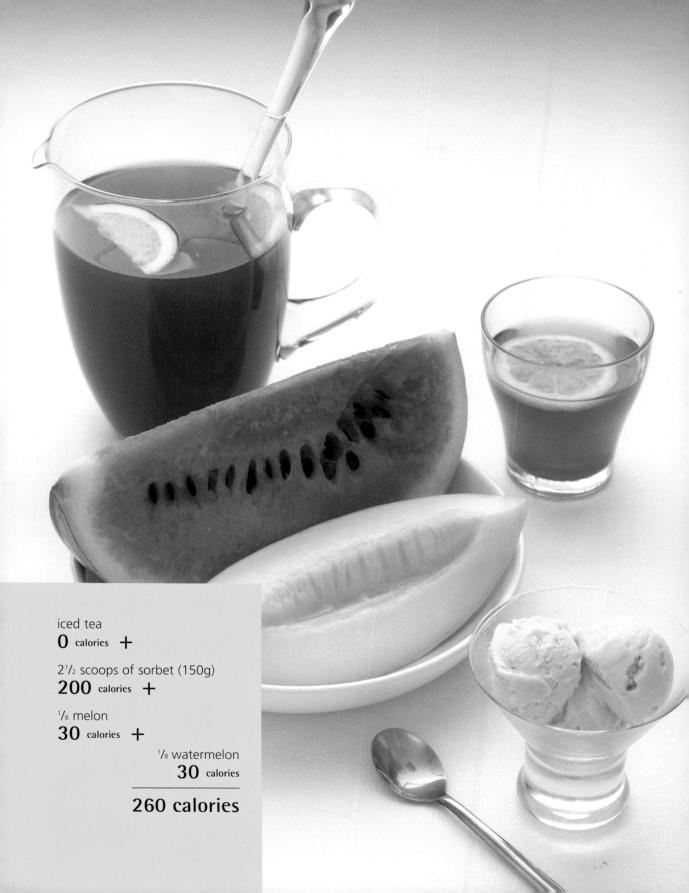

iced tea
0 calories **+**

2¹/₂ scoops of sorbet (150g)
200 calories **+**

¹/₈ melon
30 calories **+**

¹/₈ watermelon
30 calories

260 calories

THE CAROB CONUNDRUM

Carob is a classic 'food saboteur' – a food that pretends to help you lose weight. It seems nutritionally correct and bills itself as the low-fat answer to chocolate. But, in fact, carob is a substitute that has *more* calories than real chocolate – thanks to the processing that turned the carob into a snack bar. If it's chocolate you want to eat, then by all means eat chocolate.

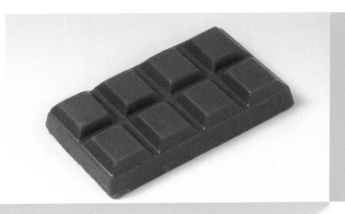

carob bar (45g)

230 calories

VS

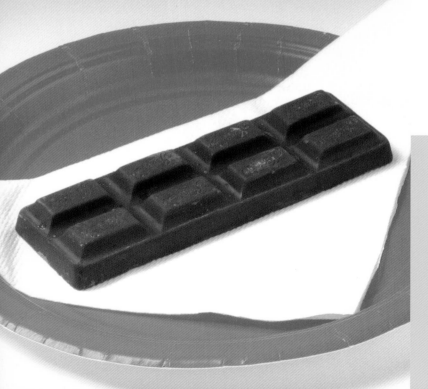

chocolate bar (45g)

190 calories

BE LOYAL TO LOLLIPOPS

Just because you're watching your weight doesn't mean you can't allow yourself a little fun. Jellybeans are a sweet treat that taste nice, but you'll polish off a handful within minutes. For the same number of calories you can suck on three lollipops, which will take you a great deal longer to eat, thus prolonging your enjoyment and leaving you triply satisfied.

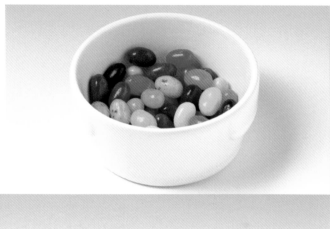

jellybeans (45g)

150 calories

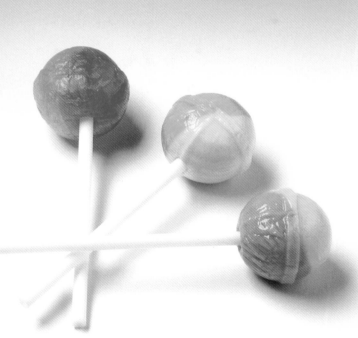

3 lollipops

150 calories

LOADS OF LOLLIES

When you crave something rich for a delicious dessert, think about getting it in a frozen ice lolly. The demonstration shown here illustrates how calorific luxury ice-cream bars can be – you can eat 10 regular ice lollies for the same sum of calories. Okay, so you probably wouldn't want to or couldn't eat 10 ice lollies, but just picture this very graphic equation the next time you reach into the freezer for dessert.

'If you've got a sweet tooth, choose your dessert carefully, and then let go of your guilt complex.'

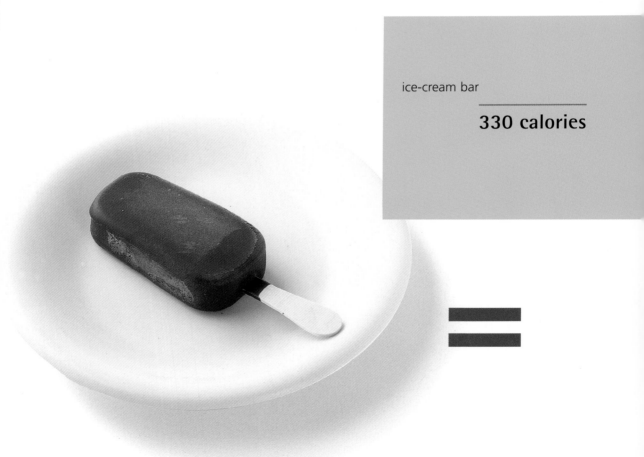

ice-cream bar

330 calories

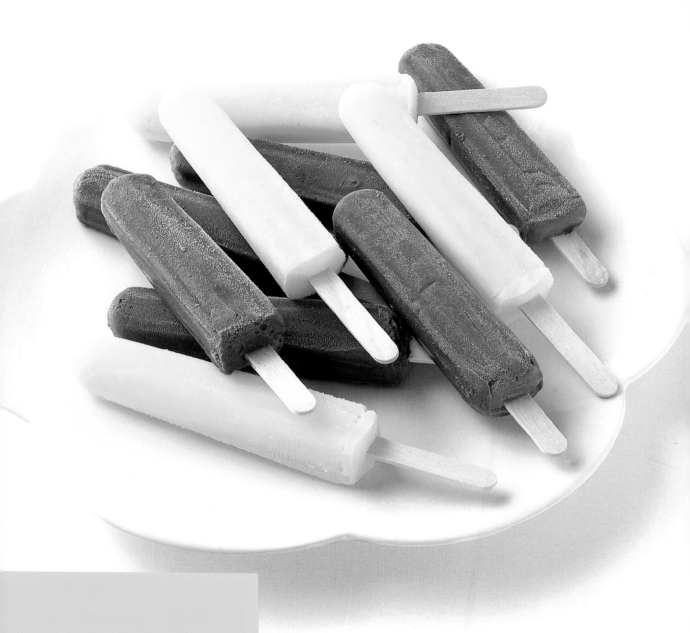

10 ice lollies

330 calories

CHAPTER 6: WEEK 3 – WHAT'S FOR DINNER?

YOUR WEEK 3 AGENDA

By the end of Week 3, you will have:
◆ Reassessed, reconfirmed and recommitted yourself to Picture Perfect Weight Loss.
◆ Learned to explore the unfulfilled needs that may influence your eating habits.
◆ Chosen a recreational activity or sport.
◆ Turned dinner into an opportunity for realising the full potential of Picture Perfect Weight Loss choices.

The family dinner is in danger of extinction. Increasingly, the typical family – say a family of four – operates on four separate schedules, especially if the children are teenagers, and that can mean four separate dinner menus at four separate times. And more and more,

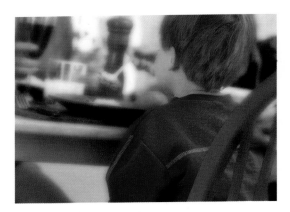

Relative values
Sitting down to eat adult-type food increases a child's experience, variety and quality of food and provides an opportunity to have a more nutritious, balanced meal.

when the family *does* sit down together, it's only briefly and rarely in a relaxed manner.

These are reasons why I'd like to make a plea to the readers of this book to reinstate the family dinner. In our culture, after all, dinner tends to be the main meal of the day.

The family dinner is in danger of extinction

Let it also be a time when the family can sit and talk. And for those undertaking the Picture Perfect Weight Loss programme, try to make dinner the meal where you demonstrate the full potential of healthy, low-calorie foods – for yourself, and for your family as a whole.

AT THE HALFWAY MARK

This chapter is about more than coming up with new answers to the classic question, 'What's for dinner?' This is because as Week 3 gets underway, you're at the halfway mark of the 30-Day Plan, and that's usually a time when people take a breath and re-examine what they're doing. Fine. Let's re-examine it together. In fact, let's make the re-examination step 1 of a five-step assignment for this week.

STEP 1: REASSESS, RECONFIRM, RECOMMIT

If you've been conscientious about your 'assignments' for Weeks 1 and 2, if you've been making new food choices, exercising regularly, filling out your food diary and paying attention to your emotional patterns of eating, then you should be well on your way to losing weight. Typically, it is in Weeks 3 and 4 that my patients tell me – invariably in a tone of surprise, if not astonishment – 'I don't even feel like I'm dieting!'

Of course, that's because they aren't dieting. If this were a diet, and you were depriving yourself of satisfying food, or weighing and measuring your portions, or telling yourself never again to eat chocolate or ice cream or cheese, then by the halfway mark, you would probably be thinking to yourself, 'I don't think I'm going to be able to do this.'

Well, you're not on a diet, not depriving yourself, not restricting portion sizes, not giving up anything forever. But you are undertaking a fundamental change in your relationship with food, and while you are certainly losing weight, you may be losing it slowly.

WE ALL MAKE MISTAKES

You may have made inappropriate food choices a couple of times. Maybe you just couldn't resist a rich and creamy dessert after dinner the other night. Or maybe you just got tired of the same salad for lunch and opted for a cheeseburger one day. So what! A cheeseburger for lunch doesn't mean you've ruined the whole day; pick up the Picture Perfect Weight Loss programme again at dinner. A single 'mistake' is all part of the learning process.

Furthermore, that single inappropriate choice is not a sign of failure to come; what you did last Thursday doesn't mean that you will make the same inappropriate choice next Thursday or a Thursday two months from now. Inappropriate food choices are not signs of a weak character, of someone who is hopelessly incapable of changing his or her relationship with food. Change isn't always a walk in the park, and Picture Perfect Weight Loss isn't even asking you to change everything – or anything – all at once. In fact, it assumes that the odd cheeseburger and occasional lavish dessert are part of life. They're not grounds for guilt or self-doubt or self-criticism.

Maybe you've been on a dozen diets in your life – maybe more. It's because they haven't worked in the long term that you're reading this book. But failed diets of the past have nothing to do with the changed relationship with food you're learning now. This is a new time, and you're undertaking a new initiative – a lifetime initiative. You're ready for change, and you've made a good

> **Inappropriate food choices are not signs of a weak character**

beginning – even with 'mistakes' and inappropriate choices. This is a process, a journey. And like any journey, it doesn't move smoothly in a straight line. There are bumps and potholes along the way. You are halfway to making Picture Perfect Weight Loss the guide to your eating habits for life. Keep at it.

WHAT ABOUT MY CHILDREN?

If your child has undertaken Picture Perfect Weight Loss, the halfway mark can be a particularly vulnerable time. After all, to kids, two weeks can seem like a lifetime. They can easily slide back into their old habits, which may look to them like a reward for the time and effort they've already spent following the programme. What's more, kids tend to lose weight more slowly than adults do, so if you're doing the programme with your kids, there may be a noticeable disparity between your weight loss – substantial and quick – and theirs. To a lot of children, this can look like failure on their part. It means that what you do at this time is even more important.

Make sure that anything you say to your child about his or her participation in the programme is positive. The halfway point is a good time to engage your child in conversation about the programme, and it's a perfect opportunity for you to review your child's own experience – to discuss the slower progress and whatever sense of disappointment there may be.

A CHILD'S EYE VIEW

In a very real sense, a child's experience with a programme like Picture Perfect Weight Loss *is* harder than an adult's. Even more than grown-ups, kids tend to measure things 'by the numbers'. It's a lot harder for them to see that success is in the actual doing, not in what the scales show. It's also harder for kids to exercise control over their food choices. Perhaps they're eating lunch in the school

> ### Be positive, proud of your child, encouraging

canteen, where the definition of 'vegetables' may not be up to the standards of their devoted mother. After school, they may find it all too easy to tag along with the crowd to the newsagents where they'll snack on high-calorie sweets and chocolate. Do you remember what peer pressure felt like when you were a kid? It's tough to resist.

Confront these difficulties when you talk to your child about his or her Picture Perfect Weight Loss progress. You might start with your own concerns by saying, 'I find

lunchtime is a real problem for me. How about you?' Let your child talk through the problem, then remind her of the changes she has made, that she's succeeding in what she set out to do, that her goal is possible. Don't compare your child to another – especially not to a sibling – nor to yourself. Be positive, proud of your child, encouraging. And be sure to ask if there's anything you can do for her, anything she needs you to get for her. Let her know that you're there to help, but be sure she understands you're not 'in her face'. Remember that, like you, kids have to undertake Picture Perfect Weight Loss *for* themselves, *by* themselves. This way it will become second nature to them.

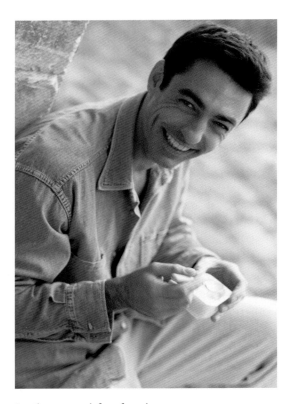

In the mood for food
Our mental state plays a major role in determining why, when and what we eat. The Picture Perfect Weight Loss programme teaches you *how* to eat.

STEP 2: WHAT'S BEHIND THE FEELINGS YOU'VE BEEN 'EATING'?

Last week, you worked at getting in touch with what you were really feeling – you learned to *feel* your feelings. In Week 3, it's time to understand the unfulfilled needs behind those feelings.

When you were 'eating' your feelings, you were trying to fill your needs with food. It didn't work; all that happened was that you put on unwanted weight. The reason it didn't work is that the need was not physiological; it wasn't really food you hungered for – it was something else. In Week 3, work on figuring out what it is you're *really* hungry for.

Start with the emotional needs we all share – the need for love and companionship; the need to succeed and be admired; the need to be productive, competent and useful. If you are wildly successful at your job and spend 14 hours a day doing it, only to come home to an empty house and a fridge full of high-calorie

> **Work on figuring out what it is you're really hungry for**

foods, chances are you are lonely – and trying to fill the loneliness with work and food. If you are perceived as sweet-natured but 'a doormat', you probably eat to make up for your lack of assertiveness. Also, it's not uncommon to find that behind a feeling of inadequacy is a fear of intimacy – both physical and emotional; being overweight offers what Dr Fink calls 'a protective barrier' against such intimacy. For adolescents, the problem is often their need for peer-group approval; if they don't get it easily, many teenagers eat instead – even though, ironically, this may lead to even more disapproval from their peers.

It's only when you know the need that you can find the right way to fill it. If it's companionship you need, for example, join a club. Take up a course. Volunteer for a community group. Wherever your interest lies, join the relevant organisation; there you'll meet like-minded people. And you can fill that need inside you – not with food, but with friends and acquaintances.

STEP 3: THE WEEK 3 FOOD DIARY

The food diary worksheet for Week 3 helps you gain an understanding of the need you are satisfying by eating. See page 114. The first two columns are straightforward and familiar. Note the day of the week, the time and what you're eating. The third column is the key, however. If you're eating a healthy, low-calorie Picture Perfect Weight Loss choice, leave the third column blank. But if you have just eaten inappropriately, your comments should prompt further exploration: are you eating without thinking? Are you eating the way you used to? If so, why are you reverting to the old habits that made you gain weight when what you are trying to do is lose weight? What need are you trying to satisfy with food? Write it down.

As always when filling out the food diary, both timing and honesty are essential. At the end of the week, when you review your diary, pay particular attention to the inappropriate choices you made. Let them help you form an understanding of your own particular psychology of eating.

STEP 4: EXERCISE THROUGH RECREATION

You've now spent two weeks exercising regularly. You started by simply moving, and last week you broadened your awareness of lifestyle exercise – and your participation in it. In Week 3, I'm going to ask you to explore a range of recreational activities so that you can find one – or more – that you can enjoy for a lifetime.

Did you play a sport at school or college? Now's a good time to take it up again. Have you always wanted to learn to play tennis? This is the moment to start taking lessons. You live alone and you like team sports? Join the local gym or visit the leisure centre. I guarantee you there's a nearby volleyball or badminton league, or a local football team. Take yoga classes. Try tai chi. Learn karate or kickboxing or Tae Kwon Do. Go bowling. Try rollerblading. Perhaps you've not been ice-skating since you were a child? Why not? Head to the nearest ice rink, lace up your skates and push away!

In other words, find something – a recreational activity that you enjoy, that you know how to do or would like to know how to do, that can exercise your body and clear the cobwebs from

> ## Take yoga classes. Try tai chi

your mind and that you can do for the rest of your life. Then start doing it – slowly, easily, only as far and as much as you can. Next week, I'll ask you to get more serious about your choice; this week is for playing around, so don't worry about your skill level or your creaking muscles. With time, you'll loosen up and improve your skills. And you will have given yourself a tool against ageing and *for* mind-clearing and energy and weight loss – for life.

WEEK 3 FOOD DIARY

Date/Time	Food (Preparation, Serving Size)	Why am I allowing myself to eat this now?

STEP 5: WHAT'S FOR DINNER? EAT THE PYRAMID

When I say 'eat the pyramid', I don't mean it literally, of course. What I do mean is that dinner is the perfect opportunity to try out Dr Shapiro's Picture Perfect Weight Loss Food Pyramid – and enjoy healthy, low-calorie eating at its best. Unlike breakfast, which calls for a particular first-thing-in-the-morning taste and texture, or lunch, which is often dependent on what's available on the sandwich shop menu, dinner is the one meal

> ## Try to fill up on protein and and high-fibre foods

you can control and your one chance to be as creative a cook as you want to be. Take advantage of it.

Most diets typically tell you to make dinner the smallest meal of the day – despite the fact that in our culture it is traditionally the main meal. Portion control like this is a mistake – in more ways than one. First, studies show that *when* you take in the bulk of your calories is relatively unimportant in terms of weight gain or loss. It's the total overall amount of calories that counts, not the hour of the day you consume them. On the other hand, 'saving' calories during the day so you can 'reward' yourself at dinner is just as much a mistake. If you deny your appetite when you should be eating breakfast and lunch, you'll be absolutely starving come dinner: you'll tend to make inappropriate choices, eat too much, and eat too quickly. The result can be the exact opposite of what you want.

So eat breakfast if you're hungry, have a substantial and satisfying lunch, and eat a snack in the afternoon if you need to. As much as possible, try to fill up on protein and high-fibre foods. They take the edge off your appetite and lower the craving for high-calorie foods. Then, sit down to dinner, relax and eat as the pyramid suggests. Turn to page 57 to refresh your memory, but here are the basic guidelines.

■ Fill up on vegetables – on their own, in salads, in soups – and fruit as much as possible. These form the base of the pyramid.

■ Get your protein in the form of soya, pulses and seafood.

■ Make grains and starches the third most important food group on your plate – and make them whole grains whenever possible.

■ Take in essential fats through olives, seeds, nuts and some oils – in moderation.

Bear in mind that frozen dinners can be a fine choice – although in my own view, most offer too little in the way of vegetables. My solution? Supplement your frozen dinner with an extra plate of vegetables or a salad or soup – or all three!

And something for afters? Choose frozen desserts – if fruit won't do. Try fat-free frozen yoghurt, sorbet or ice lollies recommended on the Anytime List (*see page 51*). Or you can always satisfy your sweet tooth with a hard-boiled sweet.

> ## YOUR WEEK 3 GOALS
>
> ◆ Remind yourself why you're undertaking Picture Perfect Weight Loss.
> ◆ Start trying to unearth the feelings you've been 'eating'.
> ◆ Fill in your Week 3 food diary.
> ◆ Try out a recreational activity – one you'll enjoy for a lifetime.
> ◆ Change your relationship with dinner by 'eating the pyramid'.

MAKE TIME FOR TUNA

Remember Dr Shapiro's Picture Perfect Weight Loss Food Pyramid? (*See page 57.*) Here's an example of just how it works. The bulk of the meal pictured opposite comes from the base of the pyramid – a couple of different vegetables with potatoes that give the meal a variety of

'When you're shopping for sources of protein, fish and shellfish are better choices than meat, poultry and dairy.'

tastes and textures, and protein from the fish. Note also that the potatoes in the tuna meal have simply been boiled, keeping the calorie count down to less than half of the potato gratin that accompanies the chops.

2 lamb chops (200g)
560 calories **+**

potato gratin (150g)
260 calories **+**

3 asparagus spears
10 calories
_____
830 calories

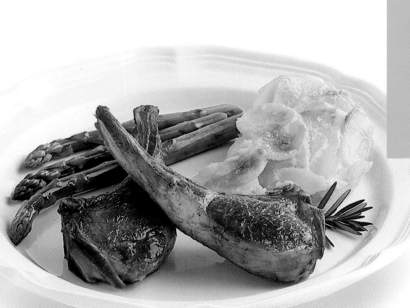

VS

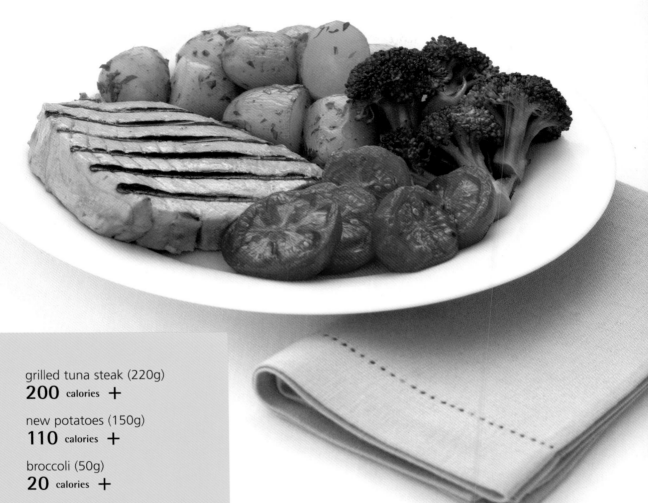

grilled tuna steak (220g)
200 calories **+**

new potatoes (150g)
110 calories **+**

broccoli (50g)
20 calories **+**

grilled tomatoes (100g)
20 calories

---

350 calories

FILL UP ON FILLET

At first glance, these two meals appear to have a similar calorie content in terms of steak. But look a little closer and you'll see that one meal contains steak *on the bone* – and therefore not as much meat as it could do – while the other consists of a prime fillet steak, meaning maximum meat content for fewer calories.

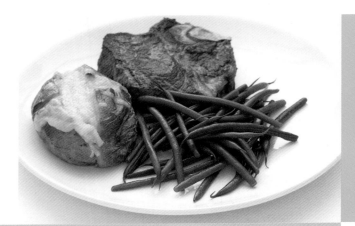

steak on the bone (250g)
500 calories **+**

large jacket potato with cheese
360 calories **+**

green beans (100g)
20 calories

_____

880 calories

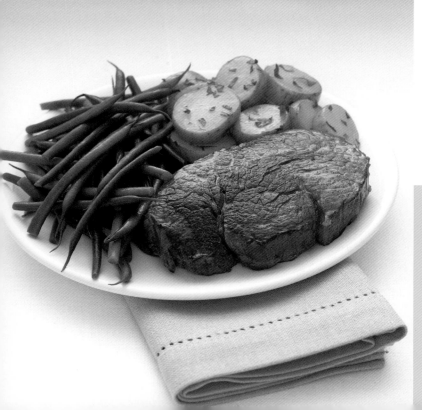

VS

fillet steak (175g)
350 calories **+**

sliced new potatoes (155g)
115 calories **+**

green beans (100g)
25 calories

_____

490 calories

THE SECRET'S IN THE SAUCE

Here are two similar Italian dishes: both consist primarily of spaghetti, both weigh 300 grams. The secret here, though, is in the sauce. The creamy carbonara sauce – containing a smattering of highly calorific bacon pieces – adds a massive 200 calories to the meal's total, whereas the tomato-based seafood dish works out at just one calorie per gram.

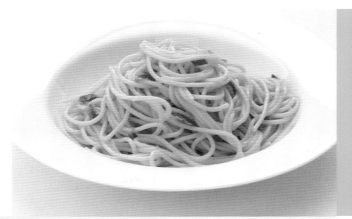

spaghetti carbonara (300g)

500 calories

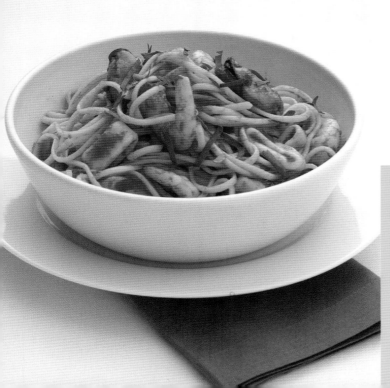

VS

spaghetti with seafood (300g)

300 calories

SCINTILLATING SCALLOPS

The spartan meal on the left looks like something someone 'on a diet' would eat on a summer's evening. Everything on the plate is low-fat, unadorned, bland. Even the dessert is low-fat, but it's also full of sugar. In fact, nothing about this meal is conducive to weight loss. It is not a low-calorie meal.

By contrast, the colourful meal on the right, with its diverse tastes and bigger portions, is a healthy and low-calorie choice. The scallops on the skewer are a better protein choice than the chicken, while the vegetables and fruit supply plenty of nutrients and will take the edge off your appetite.

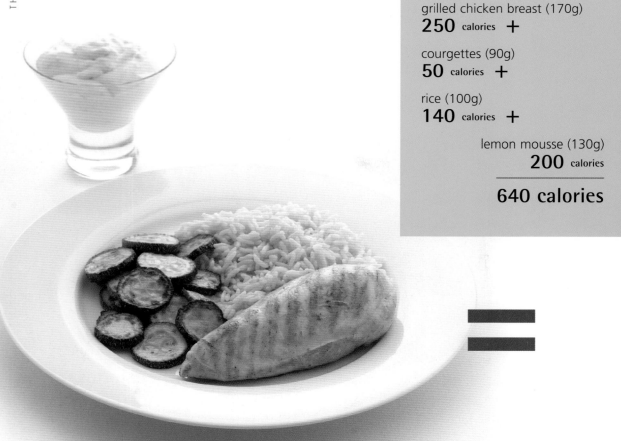

grilled chicken breast (170g)
250 calories **+**

courgettes (90g)
50 calories **+**

rice (100g)
140 calories **+**

lemon mousse (130g)
200 calories
_____

640 calories

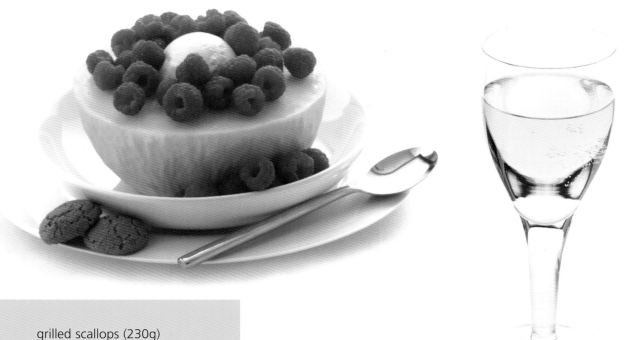

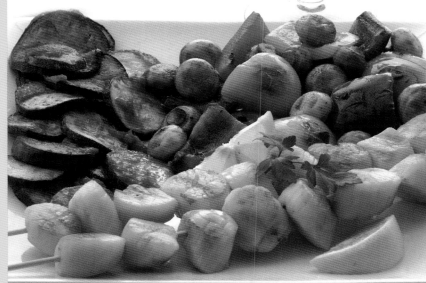

grilled scallops (230g)
140 calories **+**

mixed grilled peppers (40g)
60 calories **+**

button mushrooms (100g)
25 calories **+**

courgette and aubergine in
a herb and tomato sauce (140g)
100 calories **+**

glass of white wine (125ml)
100 calories **+**

½ melon
40 calories **+**

raspberries (250g)
65 calories **+**

2 amaretti biscuits
50 calories **+**

scoop of reduced-fat
ice cream (60g)
60 calories

---

640 calories

'Scallops are a great low–fat
source of protein and minerals.'

FISH FOR YOUR DINNER

Spare ribs are one way of getting the protein you need, but when you take in your protein through fish, you get a healthier source of nutrition and far fewer calories. Fill up on ratatouille – packed with healthy tomatoes and peppers – and enjoy French fries as an occasional treat.

'Fish is an excellent low-calorie way to eat "heart healthy" by consuming omega-3 fatty acids.'

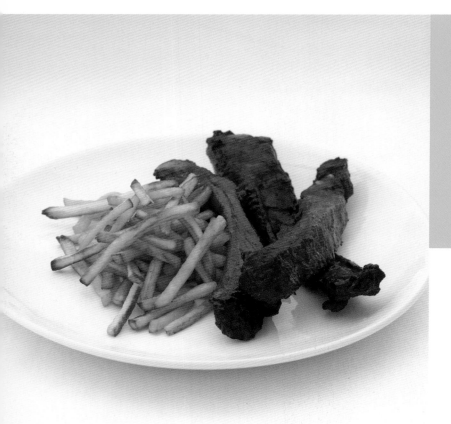

spare ribs (300g)
750 calories **+**

French fries (110g)
400 calories
_____

1150 calories

VS

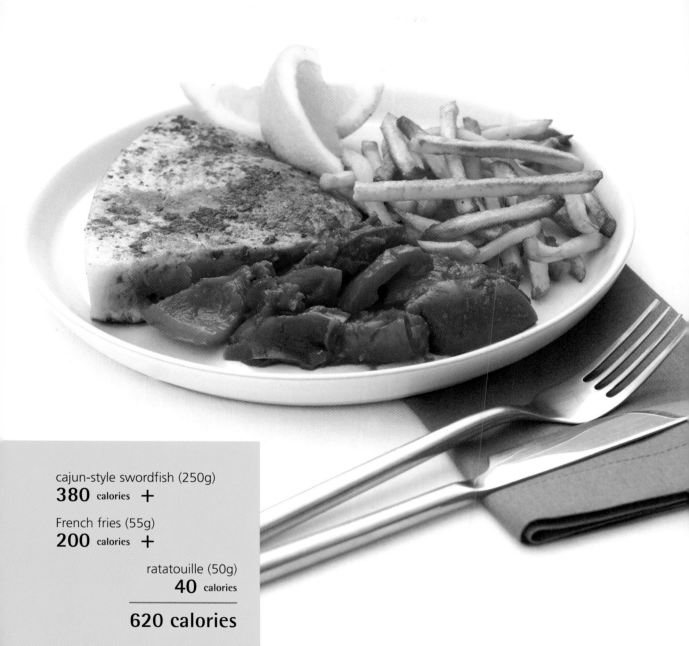

cajun-style swordfish (250g)
380 calories **+**

French fries (55g)
200 calories **+**

ratatouille (50g)
40 calories
_____

620 calories

SWEET OR SOUR?

Lemon or chocolate? Many weight-conscious people would avoid the chocolate and choose the lemon – and many weight-conscious people would be wrong. There's no calorie advantage to the lemon tart. If you're choosing it because you think you're saving calories, think again – and plunge into the chocolate cake.

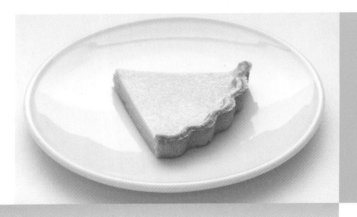

lemon tart (100g)
_____

350 calories

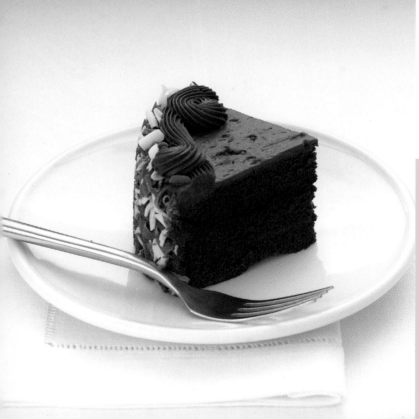

chocolate layer cake (100g)
_____

350 calories

VANILLA THRILLER

Sure, you can buy an ice-cream dessert, but how boring and calorific is that? It's just lazy eating. You're better off investing in a tub of reduced-fat ice cream, a box of wafers, a bottle of chocolate sauce – and then really going to town. Same calorific total, totally different ice-cream experience.

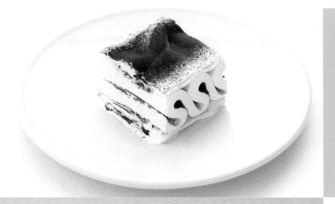

slice of ice-cream dessert (100g)

250 calories

=

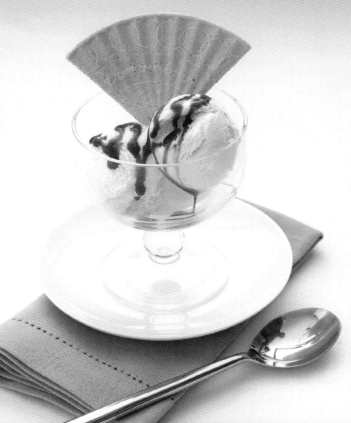

3 scoops reduced-fat
vanilla ice cream (180g)
180 calories **+**

1 large wafer
15 calories **+**

chocolate sauce (1 tbsp)
55 calories

250 calories

BLUEBERRY BONANZA

Just because you're being weight-conscious is no reason to give up the delicious taste of a blueberry dessert. However, unless you're a rugby player or a sumo wrestler, think about getting this fruit fix not from a slice of pie but from one of the seven glasses pictured on the right. Calorifically, a glass trumps a piece of pie six times over.

'Blueberries are a rich source of antioxidants – nutrients which help to keep the arteries clear and may reduce the signs of ageing.'

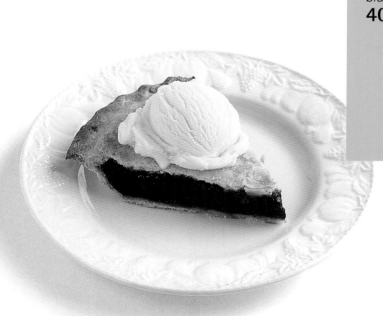

blueberry pie (150g)
400 calories **+**

scoop of ice cream (60g)
100 calories

500 calories

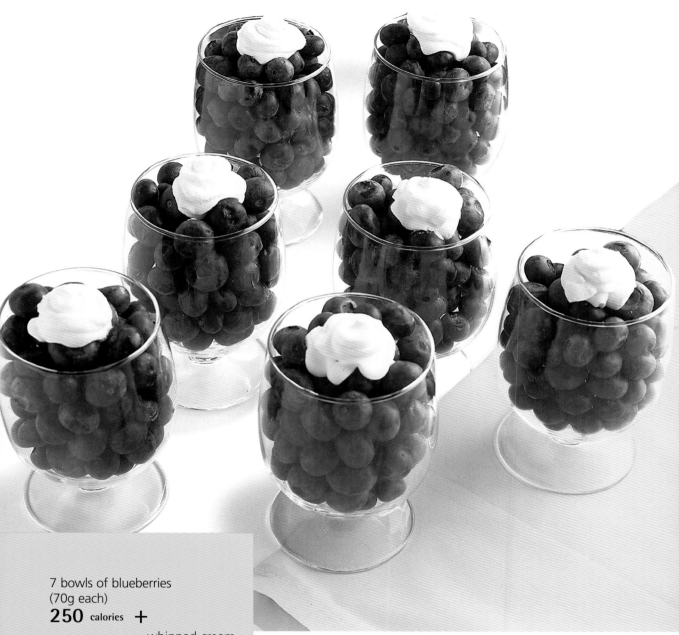

7 bowls of blueberries
(70g each)
250 calories **+**

whipped cream
(12g each)
250 calories

___

500 calories

'You can eat seven servings of blueberries for the same calorie cost as one slice of blueberry pie.'

CHAPTER 7: WEEK 4 – LET'S EAT OUT!

YOUR WEEK 4 AGENDA

By the end of Week 4, you will have:
◆ Learned how to find the appropriate Picture Perfect Weight Loss choice when you eat out.
◆ Structured an exercise programme you can follow for a lifetime.
◆ Completed your 'course' in Food Awareness Training.

THE EATING-OUT GUIDE

When you eat out, as much as you can, satisfy your appetite with generous helpings of soup, salad, vegetables and fruit. That's the key to dining out as well as the key to eating at home. Do you love the fresh bread that's served at your favourite French restaurant? Don't avoid it, but eat a smaller piece of it along with your salad or side dish of vegetables as you wait for your main course. Instead of the biggest

Go out to eat somewhere you've never been before

T-bone steak the restaurant has to offer, try a smaller cut of beef – and stuff yourself with soup, vegetables or a salad.

In other words, as I've advised before, flip the ratio. Load up on the appropriate choices and lighten up on the inappropriate choices. You'll still enjoy the tastes you love, and you'll still eat till you're satisfied.

A THREE-STEP ASSIGNMENT

It's your last full week of the Picture Perfect Weight Loss 30-Day Plan. By now, the principles of Picture Perfect Weight Loss should be almost second nature to you. Your changed relationship with food – your new way of eating – should be getting very close to being automatic. Prove it to yourself this week with a three-step assignment.

STEP 1: GO OUT TO EAT

Eat out one night. Maybe you'll choose your favourite restaurant – one you possibly haven't been to since you began the 30-Day Plan. This time, when the waitress asks if you're going to have 'the usual', surprise her by saying no and ordering something entirely new and original.

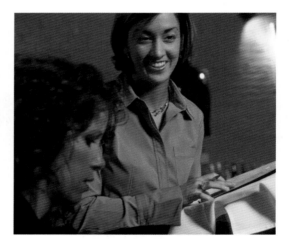

Ready to order?
Armed with the Picture Perfect Weight Loss principles you've learned over the past 30 days, go out to eat and enjoy the healthy, delicious food you love.

Or go out to eat somewhere you've never been before. It's a new menu, and you're bringing to it a fresh eye – a new way of looking at menu choices thanks to your new awareness of food and your changed relationship with it.

STEP 2: EXERCISE – MAKE IT A HABIT

Your changed relationship with food is accompanied by new habits of exercise. You've now been active for three weeks – and I'm pretty sure you feel better and look better as a result. Just think: if three weeks of basic movement can do this, imagine what a lifetime of physical activity might accomplish.

This week, make exercise a habit for life. How? By structuring a regular exercise programme for yourself. If you've thought about joining a gym, this is the week to do it. Join an exercise class or sign up with a personal trainer; for whatever kind of exercise programme you undertake at the gym or health club, it's important that you learn to do it the right way. This is particularly the case with weights or machines, where doing things the wrong way can actually prove harmful.

You don't have to go to a gym though. Maybe you've decided instead to build on the walking you've been doing for the last three weeks – to pick up the pace and lengthen the distance over time. Fine. Set a schedule. Maybe you're thinking of stepping it up a notch to jogging, or even, eventually, to running. Structure a plan. Think it through. Write it down.

Or perhaps you've decided to try yoga or tai chi. Or maybe you've decided to follow a workout DVD, or you've chosen to make golf the focus of your exercise programme, or cycling. Excellent. Remember to ease into it. Don't push yourself beyond your own comfort zone. Keep in mind that progress moves in increments. Remember that you're in this for life; don't rush it.

Please don't think I'm suggesting that you pick an activity this week and stick to that particular activity for life. Not at all. You may find that six months or a year of regular cycling on country roads, great fun as it seems at first, eventually becomes boring. The solution? Find an alternative activity. In fact,

This week, make exercise a habit for life

as you become stronger and more skilled, you will naturally seek out fresh exercise options.

It isn't a particular activity or sport or exercise programme you must commit to; it's the fact that you're exercising that's key. Just as you've established a new relationship with food, you must also establish a new relationship with physical activity. Just as you're committing yourself to a new way of eating for life, so you must also commit yourself to regular exercise for life. The specifics may change with time – *will* change, in fact, and probably *should* change – but the habit of physical activity must be an integral part of your life *for* life. Maintaining weight loss and staying healthy depend on it.

The point this week is to formalise your exercise: structure it into a programme and create a schedule. This way, you're telling yourself that exercise is an essential part of your life – and that structuring it and creating a schedule validate your commitment to it.

Whatever exercise programme you undertake, it should adhere to the following two guidelines.

Exercise regularly – and focus on it. Research indicates that even brief periods of low-intensity to moderate-intensity physical activity have weight-loss and health benefits. Still, try to work up to at least 40 minutes of exercise at a time at least every other day. Your workout should be broken up as follows:

■ 10 minutes of warm-up
■ 20 minutes of activity
■ 10 minutes of cooldown

It's also important to pay attention to the exercise you do while you're doing it. Even if 10 minutes is absolutely all you can manage today, give the activity your full attention for every one of the 10 minutes. This is your time. Make it count.

Include aerobics, strength training and flexibility training in your exercise routine. Here's a classic example: some brisk walking or cycling for warm-up aerobics, 20 minutes of weight-bearing exercise, and then 10 minutes of stretches to cool down. Of course, it's up to you to mix and match — there's nothing wrong with one day being all aerobics, the next a yoga class for flexibility, and the next all weight training.

> **It's important to pay attention to the exercise you're doing**

STEP 3: YOUR PERSONAL FOOD AWARENESS WORKSHEET

By the end of this week, you will have graduated in the Food Awareness Training course that is at the heart of Picture Perfect Weight Loss. That makes Week 4 of the 30-Day Plan a good time to create your own personal Food Awareness worksheet. It will

MY PERSONAL FOOD AWARENESS WORKSHEET

New Low-Calorie Foods (at least 10)	High-Calorie Foods (at least 6)
1.	1.
2.	2.
3.	3.
4.	4.
5.	5.
6.	6.
7.	
8.	
9.	
10.	

show you how far you've come in changing your relationship with food, and it will serve as a sign that continues to point you in the direction you want to go.

Fill in the Food Awareness worksheet any time during this last week of the programme. Think about it carefully. It looks simple, and it is, but it's a very important exercise, so don't rush it.

You really have changed your relationship with food

In the left-hand column, write down the 10 lowest-calorie foods you've incorporated into your life over the past three weeks. By 'incorporated', I don't mean just 'tasted'; I mean foods that you have made a part of your regular diet. Some may be entirely new to you. Others may be new only in the sense that they have gone from being foods you nibbled on occasionally to foods that have been truly incorporated into your eating habits – maybe you're eating more vegetables now, or more fish, or making sure you have some fruit every day, or discovering boiled sweets and low-calorie frozen desserts.

In the right-hand column, write down six high-calorie foods you believe you ought to eat less often, or find other choices for, or in some way ease out of your eating habits.

I'm not going to set down any guidelines about what should or should not be included in either column. If you think in specifics – hot fudge sundaes, the two vodka martinis before dinner – that's fine. If you think in broader categories – desserts, alcohol, fried foods – that's fine, too. It's your worksheet; it should reflect your perceptions.

If you come up with more than 10 low-calorie foods and more than six high-calorie

foods, that's also fine, but please find no fewer than those minimum numbers. Remember that you have all week to decide what should go on the Food Awareness worksheet, so take your time and think it through.

At the end of the week, when the worksheet is complete, have a good look at it. Look at the column on the left. See how far you've come over the four weeks of the Picture Perfect Weight Loss 30-Day Plan. Clearly, it is entirely possible to come up with new food choices and new ways of eating. You really *have* changed your relationship with food.

Look at the right-hand column from the perspective of that accomplishment. If the six or more foods listed here show you the dimensions of the task still ahead of you, the left-hand list is assurance that the task is eminently doable. After all, you've already accomplished an even more substantial task.

Take another look at the right-hand column. It's useful that you've written these items down. It may enhance your awareness so that the task of minimising these foods in your life or reaching out for new alternatives becomes much easier to accomplish. The list is a good thing to keep in mind whether you're at home, at work or eating out.

YOUR WEEK 4 GOALS

- ◆ Eat out at a restaurant. Using your new-found food knowledge, order the Picture Perfect Weight Loss choices on the menu.
- ◆ Decide on your choice of exercise, structure a programme and commit to your workout schedule!
- ◆ Assess your Food Awareness progress: recognise what you've accomplished and evaluate the task still ahead.

PIZZA PERFECTION

It's no secret that pizza is in no way a low-calorie snack. But if you are going to allow yourself this treat, consider the calorie difference between deep-pan pizza with meat and cheese and a thin-crust slice of Margherita. The 130-calorie difference is enough to allow you a healthy salad and a very welcome glass of wine.

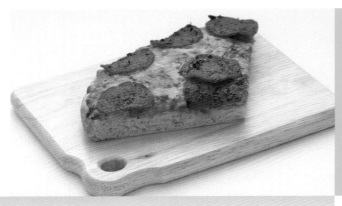

1 slice of deep-pan pepperoni pizza (200g)

580 calories

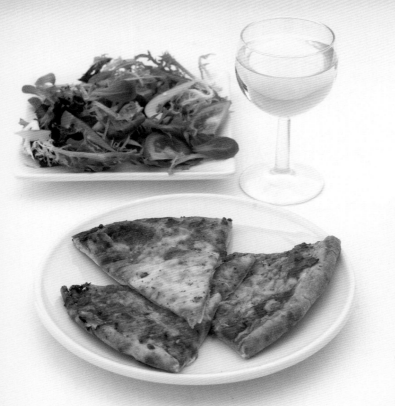

3 slices of thin-crust
Margherita pizza (200g)
450 calories **+**

salad
30 calories **+**

glass of white
wine (125ml)
100 calories

580 calories

SOMETHING ON THE GO

You're out shopping and you fancy a quick bite to eat with a beer. Once upon a time a hot dog and fries would have done the job. Not any more. Load up on a filling sushi (a great mixture of protein and carbohydrates), a bursting-with-vitamins fruit salad and a low-alcohol lager – saving yourself 520 calories in the process.

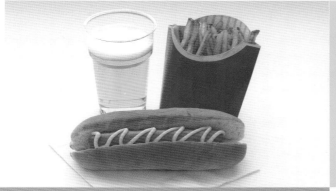

hot dog with mustard
360 calories **+**

medium fries (110g)
400 calories **+**

glass of beer (275ml)
150 calories

910 calories

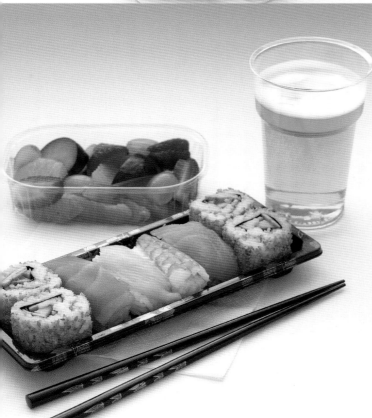

VS

sushi (175g)
220 calories **+**

fruit salad (150g)
100 calories **+**

glass of low-alcohol
lager (275ml)
70 calories

390 calories

BETTER THAN BURRITOS

Go to a Mexican restaurant, and it's all too easy to fill up on high-calorie starters like nachos or tortilla chips with guacamole before you even start on your plate of burritos smothered with cheese and sour cream. But there's a lot more to Mexican cuisine than these items. Check out the plate on the right: it's delicious, nutritious, filling and a definite calorie bargain.

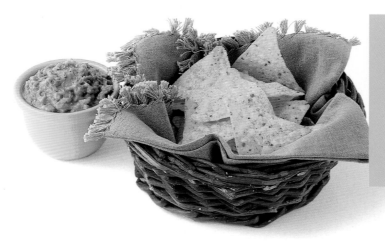

tortilla chips (100g)
500 calories **+**

guacamole (10 tbsp)
300 calories
_____

800 calories

or

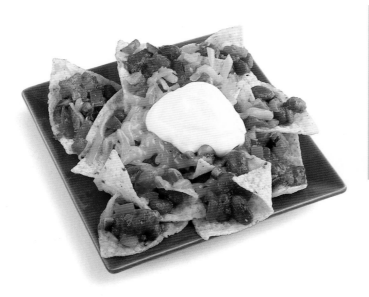

nachos (150g)
_____

700 calories

VS

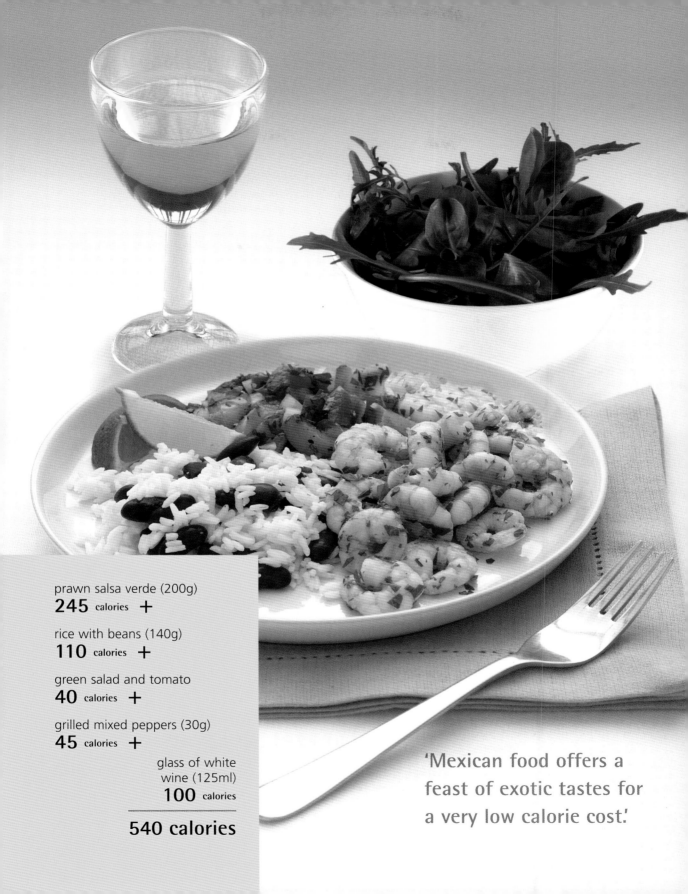

prawn salsa verde (200g)
245 calories **+**

rice with beans (140g)
110 calories **+**

green salad and tomato
40 calories **+**

grilled mixed peppers (30g)
45 calories **+**

glass of white
wine (125ml)
100 calories
_____
540 calories

'Mexican food offers a
feast of exotic tastes for
a very low calorie cost.'

A SPECIAL OCCASION

A special occasion doesn't have to be synonymous with a high-calorie meal. Take a look at this comparison. The meal on the right is every bit as impressive as the one on the left. It's also a more intriguing menu – one that is creative and that required real thought and imagination. All in all, it's a very apt offering for a special occasion – at less than two-thirds of the calories of the 'special' meal on the left.

'Deprivation? Hardly. A limited menu? Not on your life. A special occasion is still special when you eat the Picture Perfect way.'

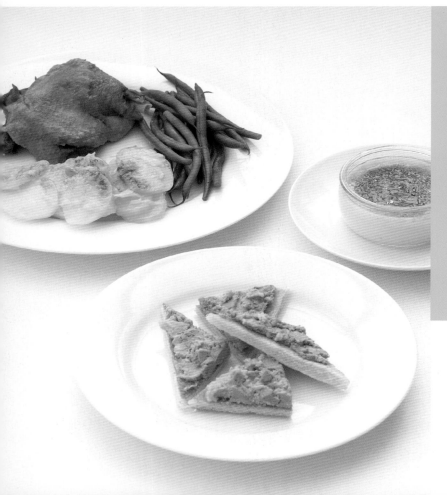

foie gras (40g) with one slice of white toast
260 calories **+**

roast duck (200g)
850 calories **+**

potato gratin (150g)
260 calories **+**

green beans (50g)
10 calories **+**

crème brûlée (100g)
310 calories

_____

1690 calories

VS

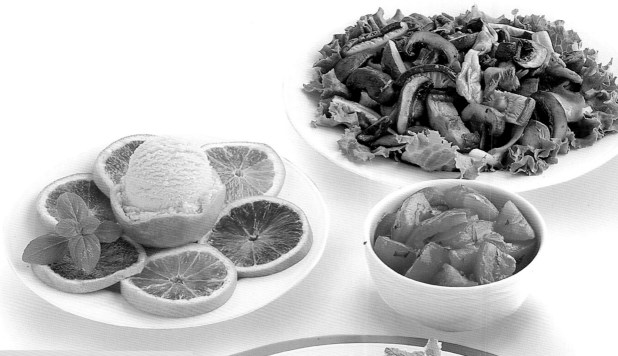

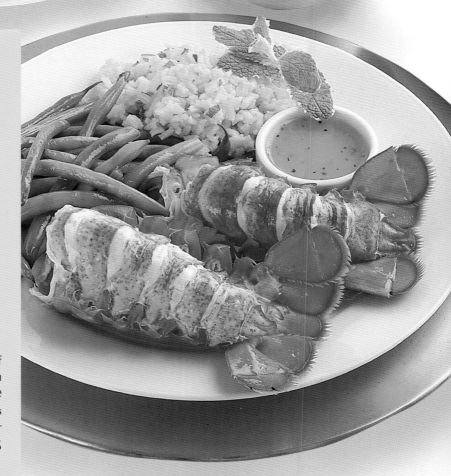

sautéed garlic mushrooms
(250g)
100 calories **+**

tomatoes with herbs (100g)
20 calories **+**

lobster tails (230g)
240 calories **+**

saffron rice (70g)
100 calories **+**

green beans (50g)
10 calories **+**

lemon dressing (2 tbsp)
50 calories **+**

one scoop of
sorbet (60g) with
½ fresh orange
100 calories

---

620 calories

CHINESE CHOICES

One of the world's great cuisines, Chinese food offers choices for a range of appetites. Some choices, however, can be high in calories – just look at these standard starters. But so much more is available that the weight-conscious should have no trouble finding alternatives. The full meal shown on the right, for example, has the calorie count of *each one* of the starters. So enjoy a full meal – and save the calories.

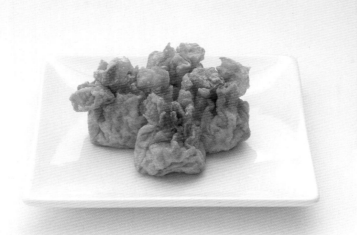

fried wontons (155g)

590 calories

or

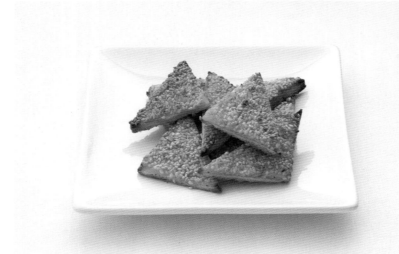

prawn toast (215g)

590 calories

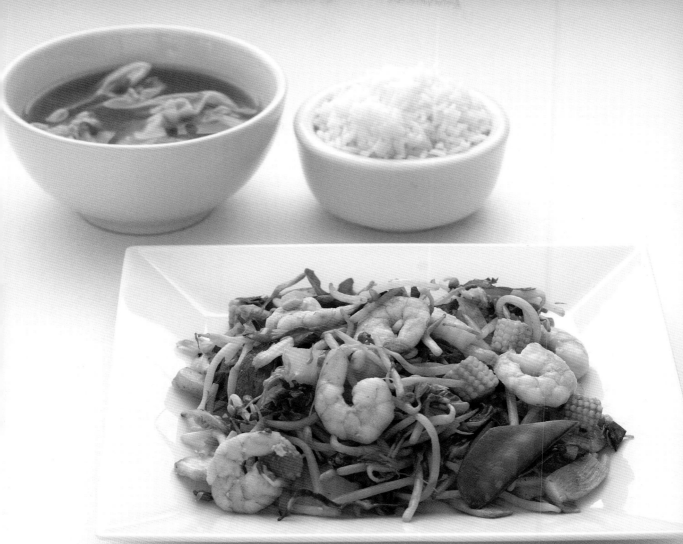

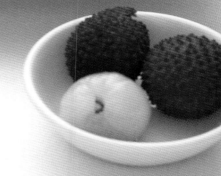

vegetable wonton soup
(200ml)
100 calories **+**

boiled rice (100g)
130 calories **+**

stir-fried prawns with
Chinese vegetables (350g)
320 calories **+**

lychees (60g)
40 calories
_____

590 calories

'A high-calorie starter or a low-calorie
meal – for the same calories.'

THE ITALIAN JOB

Many of us like to enjoy an Italian meal once in a while. However, as with most kinds of food, there's a right choice and a wrong choice when it comes to counting the calories. On the right are some alternative meal choices that give you similar quantities, similar tastes, healthier nutritional values and less than half the calories of a traditional Italian spread.

'Pasta is a treat the weight-conscious eat only rarely, so it's important to know that not all Italian dishes are created equal.'

melon and prosciutto (120g)
330 calories **+**

pasta bolognese (300g)
400 calories **+**

apple tart (150g)
480 calories

_____

1210 calories

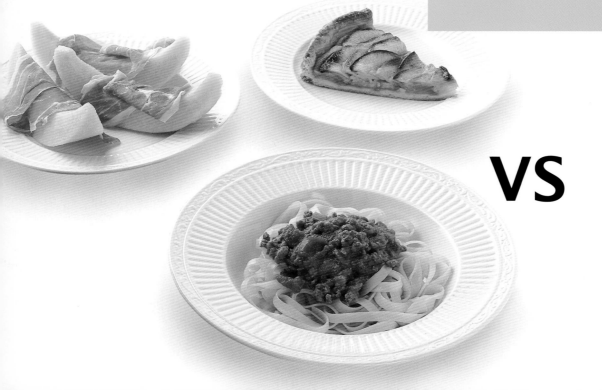

VS

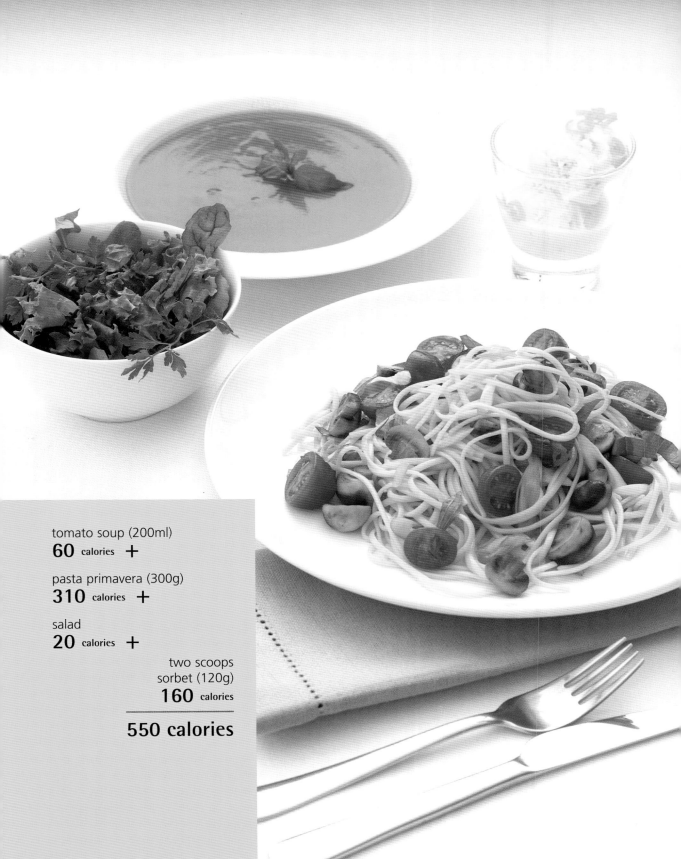

tomato soup (200ml)
60 calories **+**

pasta primavera (300g)
310 calories **+**

salad
20 calories **+**

two scoops
sorbet (120g)
160 calories
_____

550 calories

A TASTE OF INDIA

Indian food is a popular choice for eating out. The range of tastes, aromas, textures and colours is guaranteed to tantalise the taste buds. But be wary of exactly what you're ordering – or you'll pay in calories. Avoid dishes such as biryani, because they are full of cream or oil.

'Meat curries tend to have a higher fat content than veggie or seafood equivalents.'

And watch that bread choice, too; naan is often smothered in ghee, and so is high in saturated fats. A much healthier and low-calorie choice is tandoori prawns, which are marinated in spices and yoghurt. Add to this a delicious-tasting chickpea and spinach curry, and you can enjoy these Indian delicacies safe in the knowledge that you're more than halving your calorie intake.

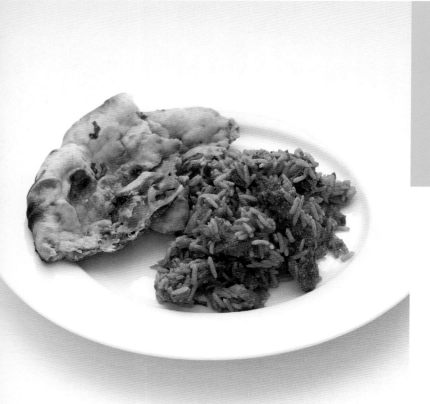

lamb biryani (450g)
800 calories **+**

keema naan (100g)
330 calories

1130 calories

VS

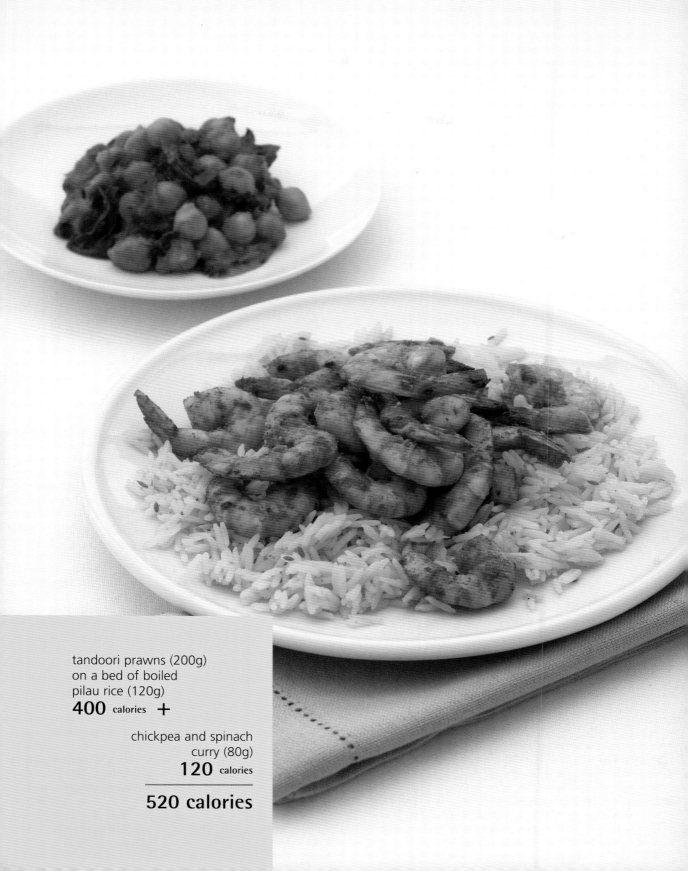

tandoori prawns (200g)
on a bed of boiled
pilau rice (120g)
400 calories **+**

chickpea and spinach
curry (80g)
120 calories
_____
520 calories

CHAPTER 8: DAY 30 – CELEBRATE!

YOUR DAY 30 AGENDA

By the end of today, you will have:
◆ Celebrated the end of the plan and the start of your changed relationship with food.
◆ Learned how to 'get through' special occasions the Picture Perfect Weight Loss way.

It's Day 30 of the Picture Perfect Weight Loss 30-Day Plan – time to celebrate. And celebrating sets the stage for focusing on low-calorie ways to enjoy all of life's happy occasions: special events, public holidays, and parties of every kind. To help with this, I'll offer tips and advice from patients who have successfully negotiated the dangerous plethora of temptations, avoiding or surviving potential pitfalls.

Before we get to the issue of eating on special occasions, there is still a little more work to do to complete our 30-Day Plan. Today, you have a simple, two-step assignment.

STEP 1: WEIGH YOURSELF

Step on to the scales, check your weight and then find the page in your personal food diary/journal where, 30 days ago, you wrote down your starting weight. Note the difference between the two numbers.

Of course, the weight loss of these first 30 days is probably not a complete surprise to you. My bet is that your clothes fit a bit more

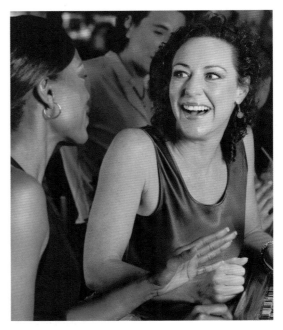

Congratulations are in order
You've reached Day 30 of the Picture Perfect Weight Loss programme. You should be feeling better about yourself in every department – physically and mentally.

loosely, your energy levels are up, and you feel better about yourself – you have more understanding of your emotional life and are more aware of your eating, more confident in a stronger body. As I said earlier in the book, this is not about numbers on your scales.

Still, seeing the weight loss measured quantitatively – seeing those numbers in black and white – can really bring home to you how far you've travelled in these first 30 days. You're in quite a different place from where you were a mere four weeks ago – and not just in terms of weight. Congratulations!

Before you close your journal, though, note also that there's plenty of room on this page to continue jotting down your weight in the weeks, months, even years to come. The point, of course, is that this first weight loss is only the beginning. You haven't come to the end of anything; you've made a successful start.

STEP 2: CELEBRATE!

At the end of fad weight-loss diets, most people celebrate by treating themselves to all the foods they've been deprived of by the diet. They'll have a blowout meal – or a blowout couple of days – filling up on those personal favourites they weren't 'allowed' to eat during the diet. That, of course, is simply the first step down what is invariably a slippery slope to regaining all the weight they've lost – and probably more.

But you're not on a fad weight-loss diet. You've now taken the first step towards permanently altering your pattern of eating and activity, and it would be a fool's errand to celebrate that achievement by reverting to your old pattern.

The fact is, though, that life is full of celebrations, and celebrations almost without exception include food and alcohol. For birthdays, graduations, weddings – from birth to death, and *including* birth and death, people the world over come together to eat and drink. You can't go through life avoiding these occasions because of a fear of having to eat high-calorie food. Picture Perfect Weight Loss is about changing your relationship with food, not your lifestyle. So how does Picture Perfect Weight Loss 'get you through' celebrations, public holidays, special occasions or even just big family meals?

You know the answer already. Your changed relationship with food keeps working whatever the occasion. It's as viable on a normal Tuesday as on the Tuesday of your 50th birthday; as practical during the dull, hard-working month of March as during the high-partying month of December. No food is forbidden, and special occasions are special occasions, but there is almost always an alternative to the high-calorie option – and now you know how to find it, and you are empowered to choose it.

> This first weight loss is only the beginning

SPECIAL OCCASIONS THROUGHOUT THE YEAR

I know: it's practically unpatriotic or a mortal sin not to overeat and overdrink on public and/or religious holidays or special occasions. Think about Valentine's Day with its promise of a romantic dinner at a fabulous restaurant, Easter with its emphasis on chocolate eggs and big meals, the hard-drinking partying on New Year's Eve. How is one supposed to 'get through' days such as these, days that almost depend on eating – even on specific foods – as integral to the way they're celebrated?

Above all, how are the weight-conscious expected to get through the food-overload of the Christmas period? For my patients and others trying to lose weight or maintain weight loss, I know that this time of year can cause a real sense of unease – even apprehension in some cases.

Of course, Christmas is typically a period of stress and anxiety as much as of joy and celebration for a great many people – those not concerned about weight loss as well as those who are. There is so much going on, so much expected of people, so much expected of the time of year itself. We're *supposed* to have fun and feel wonderful; we have an *obligation* to be happy, and that sense of obligation is the cause of a lot of stress and anxiety.

Furthermore, the party atmosphere is everywhere. There are the office parties, staff Christmas lunches . . . and then there's New Year's Eve – you name it, there's a party going on. For those who may be having a rough time emotionally, this constant round of social gatherings can simply act as a reminder of how awful they feel – and serve as another cause of anxiety.

For the weight-conscious, there's the added burden of wondering, 'How am I going to get through all the eating?' During the period between Christmas and New Year's Day, there is so much special-occasion food available on a regular basis that the issue is not so much the particular food offered at one dinner or

> ## The Christmas period can cause a real sense of unease

one party, but rather what I call the pile-up effect: the number of events at which food is the focal point and where eating and

drinking are the main activities. All of these events may be acceptable justifications for eating high-calorie food, but when you tot them all up you realise that there are more and more occasions warranting these justifications; they pile up in quick succession, day after day.

TIPS FOR WEIGHT LOSS OVER THE CHRISTMAS PERIOD

In short, during the Christmas period, both the types of food served and the circumstances in which they're served offer the weight-conscious serious grounds for concern. Still, the Picture Perfect Weight Loss philosophy remains the same – make the low-calorie choices where possible, don't waste calories unnecessarily, make sure you keep up your exercise programme, avoid deprivation, eat a variety of foods and remember that no food is forbidden. Here are some specific tips to make it easier to implement the philosophy.

You're off to a party? Don't forget to do your exercise workout first, and then eat a light snack. This will keep you from arriving at the party starved. As we know, that backfires. Take the edge off your hunger with

HEALTH TIP: ENJOY YOUR FOOD

Researchers from Sweden and Thailand have found that enjoying food is key to realising the health benefits of the food. When a simple Thai dish was served to women of the two countries, it was found that the Thai women absorbed significantly more iron from the dish than did the Swedish women, who found the food too spicy. This is evidence that the brain is the first step in digestion,

instructing the stomach to start issuing the gastric juices and thus starting the digestive process. By contrast, not liking the way a food looks or tastes can actually reduce the spontaneous muscle-driven movement of foods through the digestive tract.

Bottom line: enjoying food is important to healthy eating and to satisfying your hunger. *Enjoying* food is good for you!

a piece of fruit, for example, washed down with a couple of glasses of low-calorie drink.

Once you're at the party, keep in mind that studies show people eat more where buffet

Make the first drink a soft drink or mineral water

food is being served. Since you're not all that hungry anyway, having snacked before coming here, try to keep your distance from the food area where other guests are grazing among the hors d'oeuvres, cheeses and sausages, breads, calorie-laden dips and mayonnaise. If this is a cocktail party, remember that a meal will follow – where you should surely be able to find low-calorie choices.

Finally, a word about alcohol. There is research to support the idea that drinking alcoholic beverages may actually increase appetite. In fact, studies show that drinking prompts people to eat more, eat faster, eat for a longer time and keep on eating even after they are full. In addition, alcoholic drinks tend to be high in calories. And you probably don't need a research study to know that drinking can certainly decrease your resistance to temptation – including the temptation of high-calorie foods. So booze offers a triple whammy to the weight-conscious: it is high in calories, makes you eat more, and probably encourages you to eat high-calorie foods.

My standard advice on this subject is pretty simple – and highly effective. Make the first drink a soft drink or mineral water or even plain water – spruced up with a twist of lemon or lime if you like. Why? Because the first drink tends to go down very quickly. What my patients find is that making that first drink a glass of cool, sparkling lemonade

offers exactly the same social effect as a double whisky on the rocks – without the potentially dangerous effect on eating habits. When you've drunk it, order your glass of wine or your bottle of beer – or even better, make the second drink a soft one, too. And if the party is a dinner, ask for water as well as alcohol; then alternate between the two. It's a way to pace your drinking as well as to lessen its impact on your eating.

THE PICTURE PERFECT WEIGHT LOSS JOURNEY

Well done. We've come to the end of the 30-Day Plan – but not, as you can see, to the end of this book. What's left? Well, I've said all along that the 30-Day Plan is a way to get you started on a journey. Over the last four weeks, you've acquired the equipment you'll need for the journey: you know how to read food nutrition labels . . . how to shop for Picture Perfect Weight Loss . . . how to make different choices for breakfast, lunch, dinner and snacks . . . how to explore and express your needs. You have empowered yourself – and in the case of children, you have helped to empower your kids – to set out on an entirely new path when it comes to eating.

Like all paths, this new way of eating will have some bumps and potholes. That's what I'll be addressing in the next chapter. For now, however, celebrate! You've successfully turned onto the right road for Picture Perfect Weight Loss and a lifetime of healthy eating.

YOUR DAY 30 GOALS
◆ Weigh in.
◆ Celebrate! You're starting down a new road . . .

EATING ALFRESCO

It's a hot summer's day, and you're in the mood for eating outside. If you also want to eat a healthy and low-calorie meal, think about the choices on the right. Cool, delicious prawns with salad on slices of pumpernickel make up the core of your meal for just 250 calories. After that, fill up on bean salad, pretzels, strawberries and a glass of champagne – you won't eat more healthily for 600 calories.

'Fill up on loads of interesting and healthy low-calorie food – as opposed to high-calorie "trashy" food offering few benefits.'

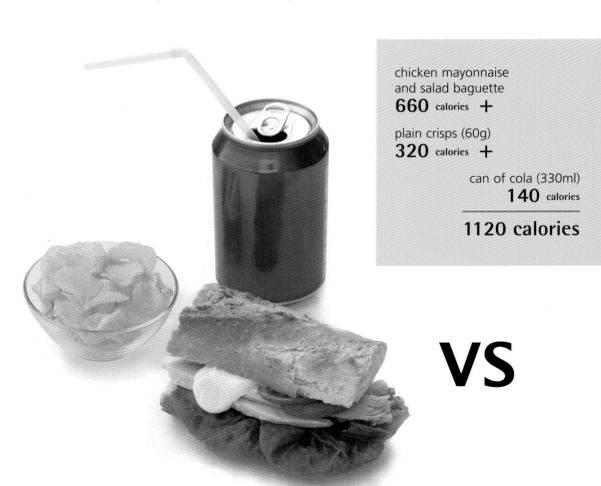

chicken mayonnaise
and salad baguette
660 calories **+**

plain crisps (60g)
320 calories **+**

can of cola (330ml)
140 calories
—————————————
1120 calories

VS

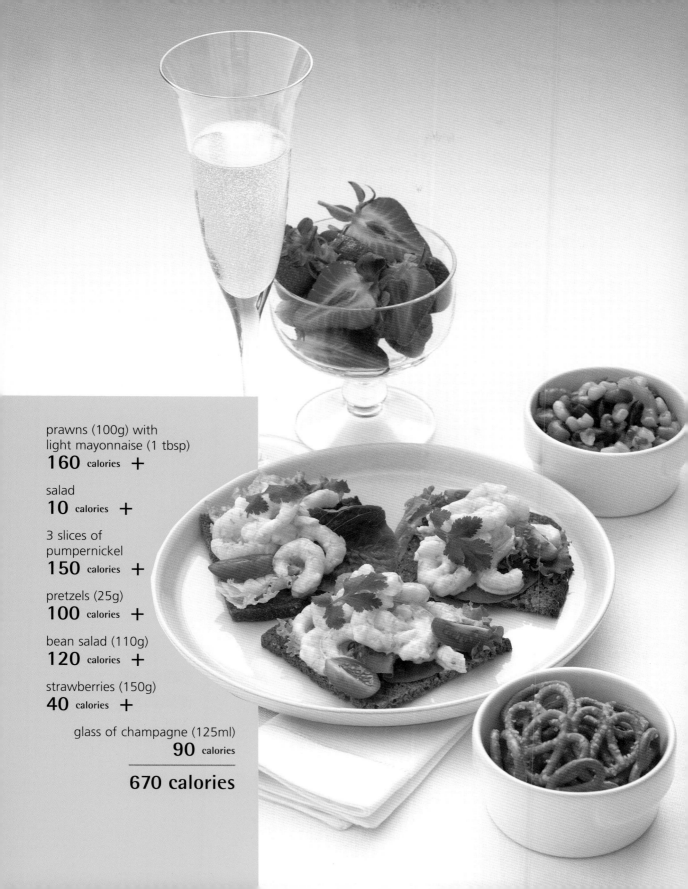

prawns (100g) with
light mayonnaise (1 tbsp)
160 calories **+**

salad
10 calories **+**

3 slices of
pumpernickel
150 calories **+**

pretzels (25g)
100 calories **+**

bean salad (110g)
120 calories **+**

strawberries (150g)
40 calories **+**

glass of champagne (125ml)
90 calories

———————————————

670 calories

THE BARBECUE BASICS

As one of my patients once said: the chicken drumsticks on the left look like the amount of food you would eat while deciding what to eat. Contrast this with the vast amount of food on the right. The lesson is simple: for the same number of calories as those meagre drumsticks, you can eat an astonishing amount of food – more varied, far healthier and much more filling food.

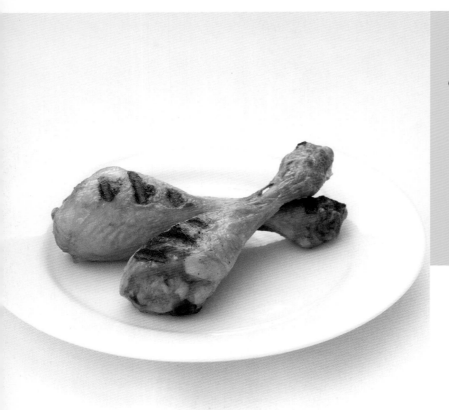

chicken drumsticks (135g)

250 calories

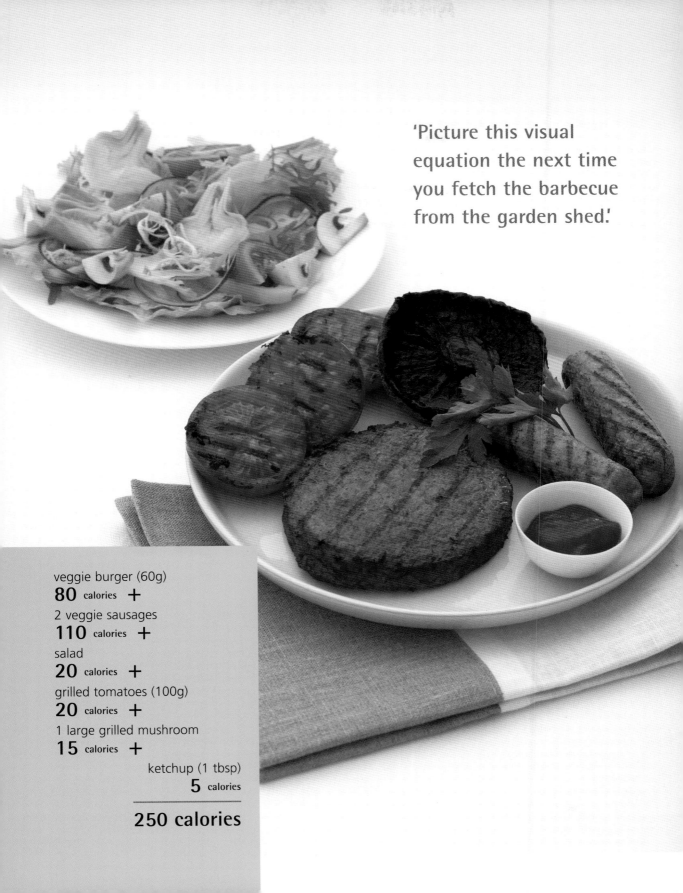

'Picture this visual
equation the next time
you fetch the barbecue
from the garden shed.'

veggie burger (60g)
80 calories **+**
2 veggie sausages
110 calories **+**
salad
20 calories **+**
grilled tomatoes (100g)
20 calories **+**
1 large grilled mushroom
15 calories **+**
ketchup (1 tbsp)
5 calories
_____
250 calories

BE AT YOUR BUFFET BEST

These quiche slices *are* delicious. And they're tempting, like so many of the foods available from buffets at parties. But before you know it, you've eaten 600 calories' worth – and you're nowhere near full! Why not opt for the cucumber, smoked salmon and capers? It will take longer to eat, it will satisfy you and it weighs in at just 300 calories.

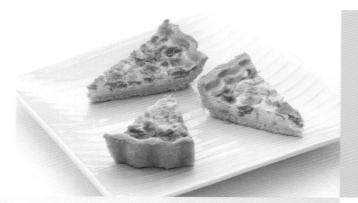

quiche slices (210g)

600 calories

VS

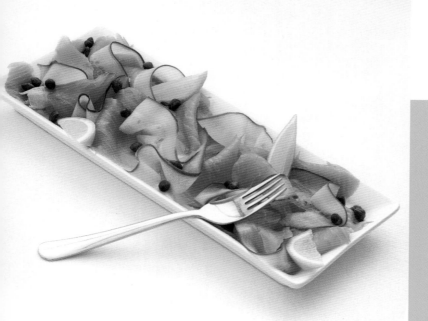

smoked salmon (210g), cucumber and capers

300 calories

CRUDITÉS FOR EVERY DAY

These springs rolls are little calorie bombs, primed to explode upon eating. What's more, they offer little real nutritional value. If it's nutrition you're after, then choose the fresh, vitamin-packed crudités selection as well as the wholemeal pitta bread. Take time to eat as you dunk them in the guacamole, hummus and yoghurt dip.

2 spring rolls (30g each)

260 calories

'Guacamole and hummus contain a good kind of fat.'

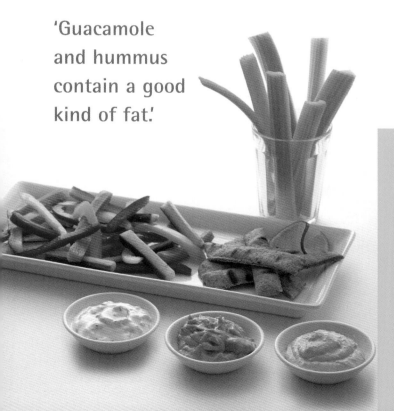

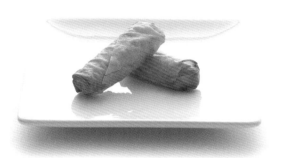

¹/₂ wholemeal pitta bread
50 calories **+**

guacamole (2 tbsp)
60 calories **+**

hummus (2 tbsp)
60 calories **+**

yoghurt dip (3 tbsp)
30 calories **+**

crudités with celery (330g)
60 calories

260 calories

THE FINEST FINGER FOOD

Finger food: it's so easy to just keep on eating it. Take the pastry snack on the left. Can you see it? It's a very small amount of food that delivers a big cost in calories. Eat the same number of calories through the choices on the right – eat all of them – and do yourself a nutritional favour while getting a jump-start on satisfying your appetite.

'Eat even a few pastry-based hor d'oeuvres, and you've consumed a substantial number of calories – before sitting down for dinner.'

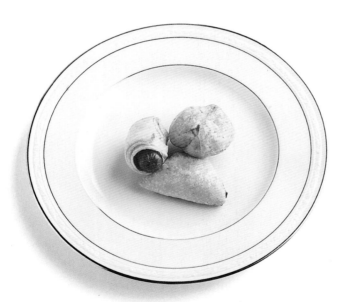

pastry-based hor d'oeuvres (60g)
_____

290 calories

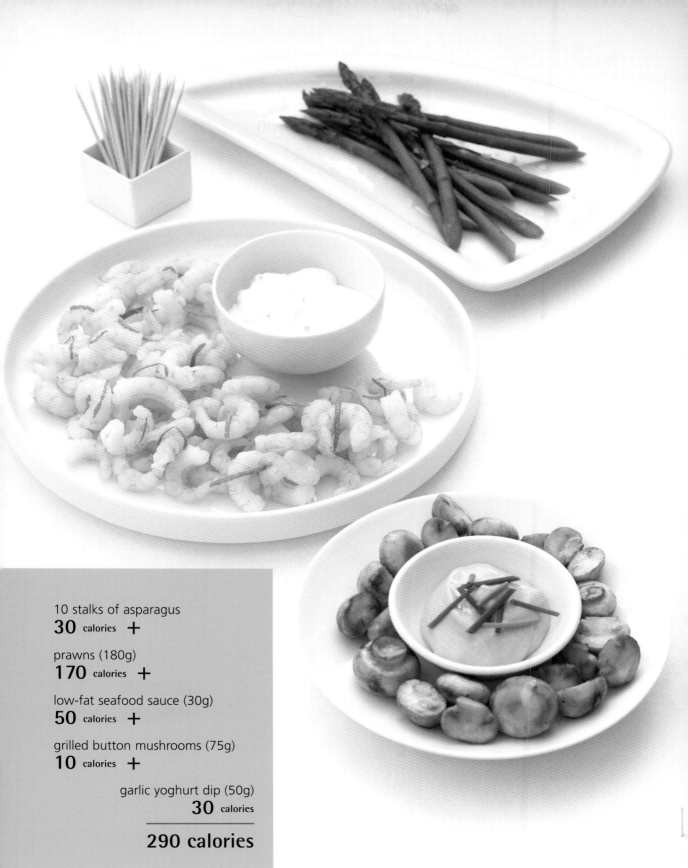

10 stalks of asparagus
30 calories **+**

prawns (180g)
170 calories **+**

low-fat seafood sauce (30g)
50 calories **+**

grilled button mushrooms (75g)
10 calories **+**

garlic yoghurt dip (50g)
30 calories
_____

290 calories

LET'S DRINK TO THIS

Of course, I'm not recommending that you drink everything pictured on the right. But just take a look at how much celebratory cheer you *could* imbibe for the same calorie count as one measly piña colada. And as we all know, the only way to celebrate is with champagne.

'The piña colada gets most of its calories from saturated fat – the bad kind of fat – found in coconut cream.'

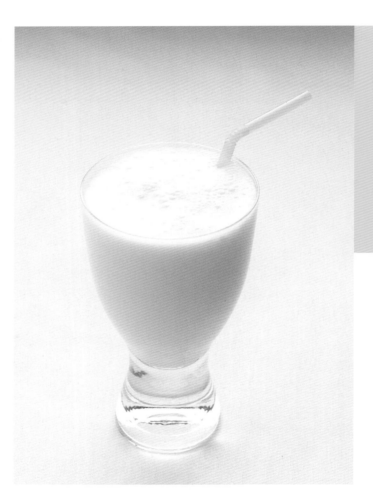

piña colada (230ml)

600 calories

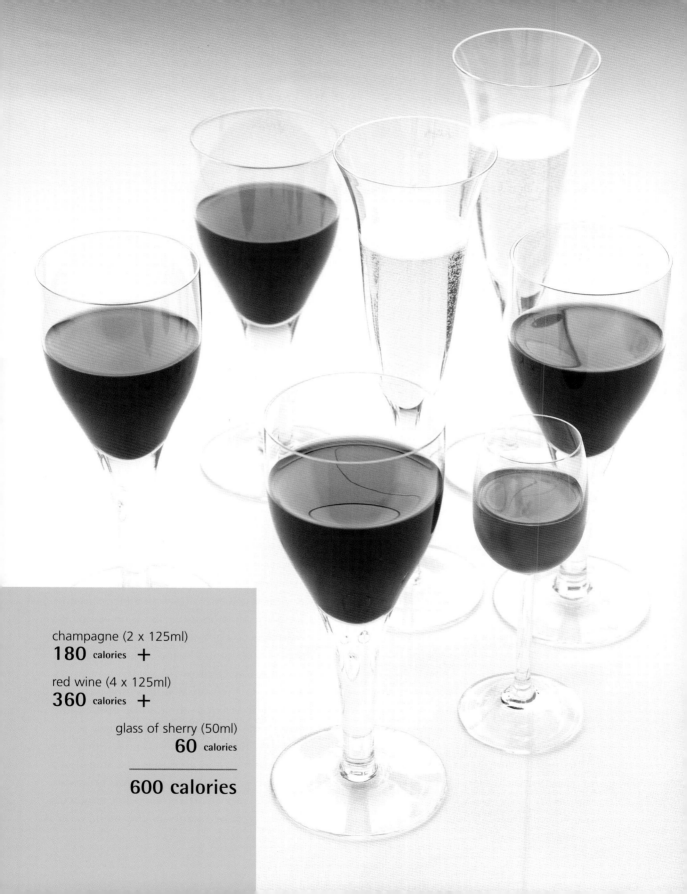

champagne (2 x 125ml)
180 calories **+**

red wine (4 x 125ml)
360 calories **+**

glass of sherry (50ml)
60 calories

---

600 calories

CHAPTER 9: THE DIET-FREE LIFETIME PLAN

I've seen it hundreds of times: a patient comes in for an appointment after a holiday of one, two, three weeks – or even longer. She 'knows' she has slipped back into old habits of eating, and she is 'certain' she put on weight during her holiday. Yet the scales shows that she has actually lost weight! A month's holiday – and she came back lighter than when she left.

Why was this patient so surprised? Why are all these patients who 'know' they've slipped so surprised? Because a holiday is outside the routine of their normal daily lives. It's time spent away, a rest – even from Picture Perfect Weight Loss! Or so you think. You're off to see new places, do fun things and experience a range of adventures. One of those adventures is eating. Whether you're heading to an exotic destination where you want to test and taste the local cuisine, or returning to your favourite resort where you know the food is superb, eating well is an integral part of what constitutes a holiday. So why didn't these patients put weight back on?

> ## You're now totally prepared to deal with all dangers

The answer is because once you have become a Picture Perfect Weight Loss eater – once you have learned the principles of Food Awareness Training and have become aware of your food choices – you never really do slip all the way back to your old habits. You simply can't.

Picture Perfect Weight Loss is a journey. There are pitfalls along the way – some hidden hazards, some all-too-obvious difficulties. Whether you realise it or not, you're now fully equipped and totally prepared to deal with all dangers; you're ready to push aside any troubles ahead. Let me show you what I mean. We'll start with some obvious obstacles.

THE SNACK ATTACK

It's 11 p.m. You left the dinner table three hours ago – satisfied with what you had eaten. You are tired and about to go to bed. But unaccountably, inexplicably, you are starving. What do you do?

Or, it's 3 a.m., and you find yourself sitting bolt upright in bed. So far from feeling sleepy, you feel an irresistible craving for something salty or crunchy. Before you know it, your bare feet have taken you to the kitchen.

Or, it's 4 p.m. You ate breakfast, had a quick but hearty lunch, and have been working flat out all day. You could do with a pick-me-up – a break for something sweet to keep you going.

How do you get past the snack attack? You don't. There is no 'wrong' time to eat. The idea that the calories in a late-night snack won't be burned off is simply not true. The notion that eating in the middle of the night means you won't sleep well the rest of the night is dubious. The theory that an afternoon pick-me-up is the first step down the slippery slope to weight gain is nonsense.

Actually, you've already started dealing with the late-night or middle-of-the-night snack.

It was back in chapter 3, when you went shopping on Day 1 of your Picture Perfect Weight Loss 30-Day Plan. What you bought then represents the food choices available to you when you're overcome by a snack attack at bedtime or in the middle of the night. For

> ## There are lots of ways to enjoy the special pleasure of dessert

that salty or crunchy craving, try a few breadsticks. If you're after something sweet, grab a couple of boiled sweets to take the edge off your appetite, or if that's not sufficient then have a fat-free yoghurt or low-fat frozen dessert.

When the snack attack occurs during the day when you're at the office, you have even more choices – and you know what to do with them. Go for a high-fibre snack like fruit to take the edge off the craving – and to fill up on your quotient of healthy nutrients.

THE DESSERT DILEMMA

To dessert or not to dessert – that always seems to be the question. And by now you know the answer: the choice is yours. Make it carefully, and if possible, go for the lower-calorie option. Remember that there are lots of ways to enjoy the special pleasure of dessert, including frozen yoghurt, sorbet or fresh fruit – all delicious, all low-calorie.

Some situations, however, make the dilemma even more problematic. Suppose you are a guest at a dinner party. Dinner was delicious, if a bit on the high-calorie side, but you filled up on the vegetables, went easy on the meat dish, avoided the cream sauce and thoroughly enjoyed your meal. Now the hostess serves a lavish chocolate cake – home-made – for dessert. What do you do?

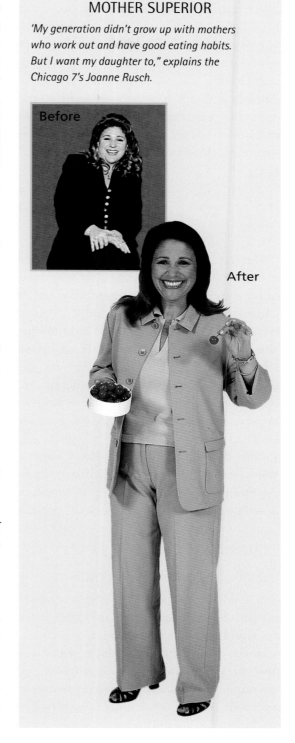

MOTHER SUPERIOR

'My generation didn't grow up with mothers who work out and have good eating habits. But I want my daughter to," explains the Chicago 7's Joanne Rusch.

Before

After

One reaction is simply to choose to have the cake because you want it. Full stop. Another is to decide it would be rude to refuse the hostess's offering – an ungracious rejection of her hard work. On the other hand, do you really want the 400 calories the cake represents? And if you have just one bite and leave the rest, isn't that just as much a rejection as saying no to the offer – maybe even more of a rejection?

Abstinence will only make the heart grow fonder

The fact is that it's perfectly acceptable and it won't offend to simply say, 'None for me, thank you,' when the cake comes your way. If you feel further explanation is deemed necessary, you have a range of possibilities. You can explain that 'the dinner was so good I have no room for anything else', or you might explain that you're 'allergic to chocolate' (yes, you react by gaining weight), or you could just say that you're 'watching the calories'. People understand.

With dessert, as with every food, rigidity won't work, and abstinence will only make the heart grow fonder. Don't be afraid of dessert. Approach your dessert options carefully – then choose the one that's right for you.

HAVE A HAPPY HOLIDAY

You're off to Paris, and there's no way you're not going to sample the culinary highlights of the world's most famous cuisine.

Holidays are a time to indulge yourself, a time to splurge. But indulging yourself and splurging don't necessarily mean reverting to old habits of eating. A holiday is a change of routine, but it doesn't mean a change in the Picture Perfect Weight Loss philosophy. It's always possible to experience the special tastes of a holiday within the framework of Picture Perfect Weight Loss.

My advice? It's simple. Pack your bags with a plan in mind. Just as you think about how you'll spend your time, consider also how you'll spend your calories. Just as you lay out different clothes to pack for different types of weather and various occasions and events, try to lay out where you might splurge on high-calorie food choices and where you can indulge in lower-calorie choices. Thinking about it ahead of time can at least take the sting out of the high-calorie choices when you confront them. Whatever you do, don't leave to go on holiday telling yourself you 'can't have' certain foods. There's no point in going to Paris to avoid croissants, is there? You're not avoiding anything; you're just planning where those certain foods will fit in.

DOWN IN THE DUMPS

Sometimes, life throws bad things at you. It happens to everyone, and whatever it is – trouble at work, relationship issues, illness, a death in the family – it can bring you down. The negative emotions increase your need to eat. This isn't an abstract metaphor. The mind and body are connected, and that's how the connection works: agitation in the mind stirs cravings in the appetite.

There's not much you can do about this, and certainly it's tough enough trying to deal with the issue that's troubling you without worrying about what you're eating as well. But just by being aware of the potential for eating without thinking, you bring the principles of Picture Perfect Weight Loss to the front of your brain – and that's where they'll do the most good in influencing your eating choices. It's important to try to keep in

HIDDEN HAZARDS: SABOTEUR FOODS

In addition to the obvious difficulties along the Picture Perfect Weight Loss path, there are also hidden hazards. Among the most potentially damaging of these hazards are saboteur foods. These are foods that pretend to help you lose weight. But the fact is, these foods serve no purpose in weight control. They are the high-calorie/empty-calorie foods that we give ourselves permission to eat because they are lower in fat or sugar than their 'normal' food counterparts.

All too typically, when we give ourselves permission to eat these foods, we can easily rationalise overeating them. That is why saboteur foods are the only foods I suggest you avoid in my weight-loss programme. Quite simply, they will sabotage your weight-loss efforts and undermine the results.

High on the list of saboteurs are low-fat and fat-free baked goods. To read the advertising on these products, you'd think weight would vanish in an instant. The evidence – and there's lots of it – shows otherwise. All you're really doing is exchanging one kind of calorie for another.

There are many other saboteurs besides these obviously misleading (and oh so tempting) baked goods. In fact, I divide saboteur foods into two main categories: the have-nots, and the haves.

The have-nots are all those snack foods with advertising that lists all the 'bad' ingredients they do not contain. They are low-fat, reduced-fat, sugar-free, low-sodium and so on. The no-cholesterol claim is the one that really gets my goat. Cholesterol-free foods can still be high in ingredients that really add weight. Crisps and chips, for example, have no cholesterol, but they are loaded with fats and are very high in calories.

The other category of saboteur foods – the ones I call haves – are the ones I refer to as 'healthy naturals'. We mistakenly perceive these foods as having some redeeming nutritional benefit.

Maybe the product is sweetened with fruit juice or honey instead of with refined sugar. Or the snack bar is made of carob instead of chocolate. Perhaps the crisps are made from vegetables other than potatoes. The list goes on and on. The replacement item sounds healthy and natural, so we rationalise that it isn't as bad as an empty-calorie food.

But a biscuit sweetened with honey is just as high in calories as one sweetened with sugar. And crisps made from sweet potatoes or parsnips, instead of from regular white spuds, differ from traditional potato crisps only in content, not in calories. They're not any better for you. So don't eat them.

mind that high-calorie food won't put an end to your troubles or lift you out of your depression. In fact, the mind-body connection can work both ways, so that healthy, low-calorie eating may have as real an effect on your mind as your mind has on your body.

Of course, so can exercise, and this might be the time to try physical exertion as a new approach to the blues. Research has shown, for example, that a 'runner's high' doesn't happen only to long-distance runners. Sustained, focused exercise affects certain neurotransmitters in the brain for a kind of 'natural Prozac' effect. Besides, it can take your mind off your troubles.

FEAR OF THINNESS

Even harder to discern among the potholes that can trip you up on the path to Picture Perfect Weight Loss is the sheer fear of thinness. What makes fear of thinness so hard to see is that it is rooted in an individual's psychology – and it can take many forms. Yet

> ## Change – in the form of losing weight – can be scary

all of the guises in which fear of thinness appears have one underlying similarity: the thing that is frightening is the change from being overweight to being thin.

There are no two ways about it: change can be scary – both to the person effecting the change and to those around him or her. It can seem threatening; it threatens to disrupt a way of life that, for good or bad, has become comfortable, manageable, understandable. People resist that sort of disruption – often unconsciously. Amazingly, even the person who wants to be thin can find himself or herself resisting becoming thin.

ROCKING A RELATIONSHIP

Picture Perfect Weight Loss may change the dynamics of your relationship with your spouse or lover, children, friends and colleagues. In many cases, as my staff psychotherapist Susan Amato puts it, 'a person who is overweight serves a purpose in a unit – that is, in a couple or family. When one person in the unit loses weight, the whole unit changes.' You don't want to, but you may inadvertently rock the boat a little.

STAND UP FOR YOURSELF

'I never understood the concept of "toxic people". But I would often find myself with such people, and I see now how I used to give into them, go and eat something and then feel powerless. Now I just choose not to be in their company,' says Heidi McInnery, a member of the Chicago 7.

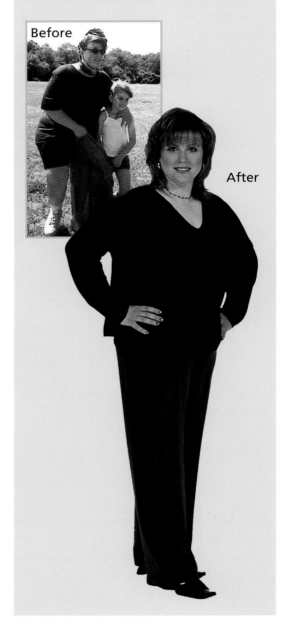

Before

After

Children who were used to a cosy, comfortable, chubby mum may find a svelte, glamorous mother unsettling. Readjustment can take time.

A husband or wife may suddenly — and unconsciously — feel insecure about the other's weight loss. Maybe he or she fears it makes the spouse attractive to the opposite sex in a new way — and that makes him or her vulnerable in a new way. It sounds far-fetched, but the worried spouse may even try to sabotage the other's weight loss — maybe by bringing home 'gifts' of chocolate or sweets, or by urging that the weight loss be 'celebrated' at a lavish restaurant, where high-calorie foods are pushed under the nose of the newly thin partner.

Even friends may be threatened by your weight loss. For one thing, the overweight person is often the unthreatening 'universal mate' who is invited to everything. He or she is typically thought of as an easy, unassuming presence — one who's not going to snare a

> ### Picture Perfect Weight Loss is your decision – do it for you

member of the opposite sex, for one thing, but also someone who can always be relied on to fill the numbers, show up and listen to everybody else's tales of woe.

Lose weight, and your friends start to assume the weight loss has affected your character. 'Can I still rely on her?' they may wonder. 'Is she now going to be a threat to me when we're out for the evening and we talk to guys? Didn't she used to be more fun — back when she was overweight and jolly?'

As the dynamics of these relationships begin to shift, even the person trying to lose weight may hesitate. Consciously or unconsciously, you may feel a reluctance to 'disappoint' your children, worry your spouse, unsettle your friends. If so, stop! Picture Perfect Weight Loss is your decision; you're doing this for *you*, not for others. Their needs are their responsibility. Your responsibility right now is to you — to your need to lose weight, even if it means change. Good friends and most partners will appreciate you getting control of your life — and delight in the hitherto undiscovered part of your personality. After all, while it may be a cliché to say so, variety *is* the spice of life. Finding new aspects to a relationship can be exciting — even if it might seem a bit unsettling.

FEAR OF INTIMACY

It's not only your effect on others that you may worry about as you lose weight; you may also have to confront some deep-rooted worries of your own, worries that being overweight had kept undercover. Psychologists often talk about the 'secondary gain' that some people get from problems that seem, on the surface, to be really disturbing to them. The secondary gain that many overweight people experience is a protection against intimacy. After all, being overweight can take you out of the dating game, can serve as a barrier against the 'messiness' of a romantic relationship, can take you out of the running for marriage or a lover or sexual activity. Phew! Now you don't have to compete, take a risk or maybe get rejected. What a relief! Sex ceases to be an issue; even your own sexual appetite can simply be repressed, hidden away beneath your weight.

Not surprisingly, for some people, weight loss can regenerate all those fears of intimacy that have been allayed for so long by being overweight. It's one of the key reasons these people resist weight loss, even though they know somewhere inside themselves that they want to be thin.

Unfortunately, there's no avoiding the risks of intimacy – and no substitute for intimacy's rewards. Relationships with others are messy, but they're worth the effort. Burying the possibility of intimate relationships by being overweight works only up to a point; if it were really making you happy, you wouldn't now be undertaking Picture Perfect Weight Loss. Stick with it. It will open up a whole new, exciting world that you will now have the courage to enter.

FEAR OF EXPOSURE

Fear of thinness really comes down to fear of exposure. It's the fear of receiving attention, the fear of how others perceive you, the fear of being seen through, the fear of having to compete with everyone else – a kind of performance anxiety. It makes people uncomfortable. Remaining overweight is so much safer.

In fact, remaining overweight can be an eternal excuse: you didn't get that last job promotion? It wasn't your job performance; it was your weight, you reason. Someone else got the part in the play? You console yourself with the thought that it wasn't that you have no talent; it was that you didn't 'look the part' – that is, you weren't thin enough.

A delightful patient from a few years ago was an opera singer, a job in which being overweight is not traditionally considered a shortcoming. Yet Sharon never got the good jobs, never did well in auditions. 'It's because of my weight,' she kept insisting. But the truth was that Sharon's voice, although pleasant, didn't have the power or range or distinctiveness that her chosen field demanded. And as long as she remained overweight, she avoided facing that truth.

Sure enough, as Sharon lost weight, she had to come to grips with the fact that she wasn't going to make it as an opera singer, not because of her weight, which was now no

Fear of thinness really comes down to a fear of exposure

longer an issue, but because she really didn't have what it takes. It was a tough lesson, but having learned it, a new, thin Sharon was eventually able to get on with her life. She has changed careers, and for the first time in her life, she really feels successful.

PICTURE PERFECT WEIGHT LOSS FOR LIFE

Mike Carter, an official from New York's Uniformed Firefighters Union, lost 36kg (5st 10lb) as a result of changing his eating habits to follow the principles of Picture Perfect Weight Loss. At the time of writing, he has kept the weight off for two years.

Policewoman Dorothy Jackson, who first came to me in 1995 after her second pregnancy pushed her weight up to 77kg (12st 12lb), went down to 53.5kg (8st 6lb) – and has stayed at this weight ever since.

The Chicago 7 have lost a total of 128kg (20st 2lb) as this book goes to press; all continue to lose weight as they continue to make Picture Perfect Weight Loss their eating norm.

None of these people have changed their lives. What they have changed is their relationship with food and their eating habits. They have made changes in understanding, mindset, knowledge. Additions to the mental menu are the kinds of foods they think about eating. They have flipped the ratio. Little changes have made a big difference to all these Picture Perfect Weight Loss veterans.

BE PATIENT

'I find it easy now to run for a bus, and I can dash up the four flights of stairs to my flat,' says David Taylor, one of the patients who came to see me at my New York practice. 'I feel healthier not just in my body, but in my mind, too,' adds David.

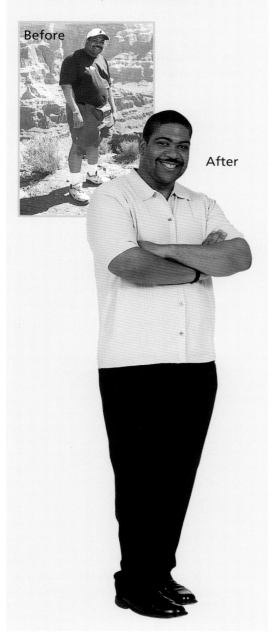

Before

After

I'm not asking *you* to change *your* lifestyle, either. What I am doing is changing your relationship with food, and asking you to make this change an integral part of your life. How will you do it? One meal at a time.

For Mike Carter, as for the firefighters he works with, the Chicago 7, and the thousands of patients I've treated successfully, *Picture Perfect Weight Loss has become a habit. Not a programme, not a project, not a special event. It's a way of shopping for food, cooking and eating that has become a way of life for these people. It's a long-term success story.*

COMMITMENT TO CHANGE

You chose to buy this book and to undertake Picture Perfect Weight Loss. You chose change. And deep down, you understood that it was a choice for life.

Are you committed? You've spent 30 days making changes. Some of the changes have been small, some big. You've introduced new foods into your daily menu and new physical activity into your weekly calendar. You've also introduced new thinking into your brain: you have new attitudes towards old foods like dairy products and recent innovations like soya-based products; you have a new awareness about calories and nutrition. You've even let yourself deal with some emotional issues concerning your view of yourself and your needs – and maybe you've begun to exorcise some old demons.

It certainly sounds like you've made a commitment. In fact, when you think about it, you've done a lot, and you've come a long way. Ahead of you is the big prize: the new, trim you – looking good, shopping for a new wardrobe, feeling energetic, choosing a gorgeous selection of low-calorie, healthy, nutritious foods day after day for life. My prescription? Don't stop now.

CONVERSION CHARTS

These equivalents have been slightly rounded to make measuring easier.

VOLUME MEASUREMENTS

METRIC	IMPERIAL
1ml	–
2ml	–
5ml	–
15ml	–
30ml	1 fl oz
60ml	2 fl oz
80ml	3 fl oz
120ml	4 fl oz
160ml	5 fl oz
180ml	6 fl oz
240ml	8 fl oz

WEIGHT MEASUREMENTS

METRIC	IMPERIAL
30g	1 oz
60g	2 oz
115g	4 oz ($1/4$ lb)
145g	5 oz ($1/3$ lb)
170g	6 oz
200g	7 oz
230g	8 oz ($1/2$ lb)
285g	10 oz
340g	12 oz ($3/4$ lb)
400g	14 oz
455g	16 oz (1lb)
1kg	2.2lb

LENGTH MEASUREMENTS

METRIC	IMPERIAL
0.6cm	$1/4$ inch
1.25cm	$1/2$ inch
2.5cm	1 inch
5cm	2 inches
11cm	4 inches
15cm	6 inches
20cm	8 inches
25cm	10 inches
30cm	12 inches (1ft)

CALORIES TO KILOJOULES (kJ)

Calories x 4.186 = Kilojoules

CALORIES	KILOJOULES (kJ)
1	4.186
10	41.86
25	104.65
50	209.3
75	313.95
100	418.6
200	837.2
300	1255.8
400	1674.4
500	2093
600	2511.6
700	2930.2
800	3348.8
900	3767.4
1000	4186

INDEX

Boldface page references indicate boxed text and tables.
Italic references indicate photographs.

ACKNOWLEDGMENTS

Many of the people who helped make the Picture Perfect Weight Loss 30-Day Plan a reality appear in the pages of the book – some of them in its photographs. But many more people were involved in the effort, and I am glad to acknowledge them here.

Thanks, above all, to Phyllis Roxland for guidance on non-meat eating and on the food demonstrations. Roz Siegel, my editor at Rodale Press in New York, and Aaron Brown at Studio Cactus in the UK provided wisdom, expertise and humour in shepherding the manuscript through to its completion. I am grateful also to Susanna Margolis, my editorial collaborator, who possesses an uncanny ability to translate my thoughts into clear and compelling language. And Mel Berger, my agent at the William Morris Agency, remains the 'godfather' of my book writing. Everyone assures me that with Mel, I am 'well looked after'. Everyone is absolutely right.

To the editorial teams in the UK who are primarily responsible for the book you hold in your hands, I offer my sincerest thanks. To the Cactus team – book designer Dawn Terrey, home economists Denise Smart, Penny Stephens and Philippa Vanstone, dietician Sue Baic and photographer Iain Bagwell – please accept my thanks for the hard work and the superb results. To the Rodale UK editorial team of Anne Lawrance, Maggie Ramsay, Helen Evans, Susannah Webster and Keith Bambury, to production guru Sara Granger and to Jane Tappuni, senior international sales manager, please accept my gratitude and best wishes.

Food stylist Diane Vezza and her assistants Joan Parkin and Rose Holden, and photographer Kurt Wilson and his assistant Troy Schnyder brought to life with great style the wonderful demonstrations that tell the Picture Perfect Weight Loss story so vividly, supplemented for this edition by Iain Bagwell's fine work. Book designer Christina Gaugler dealt cheerfully, on this book as on its predecessor, with my questions and suggestions and created a uniquely user-friendly book for users of all ages.

Those Rodale staffers who laboured in the editorial and research vineyards of the 30-Day Plan – Jennifer Bright, Lois Hazel and Carrie Havranek – added incalculable value.

Nor can I say enough about Mary Lengle of Rodale; Vanessa Menkes, Kara Cohen and Judy Drutz of Dan Klores Communications; and Jo Marshall of Midas Public Relations in London. Together, they are surely the most creative, effective and supportive publicity team in the history of the world.

I'm also grateful, on this book as on the original, Picture Perfect Weight Loss, to my friend Anne-Laure Lyon, fashion stylist, for her vision, direction and expertise.

Thanks as always to the staff at my New York office, who somehow make it possible for me to pursue two busy careers simultaneously – one as physician, one as author. Gerri Pietrangolare and Alexandra Lotito keep the office running smoothly, and nutritionist Sharon Richter, M.S., R.D. and physical therapist Les Koch provide essential services to my patients.

Special thanks to psychologist Adele Fink, PhD, who shares my office space in New York and generously shared her considerable knowledge of the psychology of weight loss. And to my staff psychotherapist Susan Amato, C.S.W., who served as counsellor to the Chicago 7 and provided substantial input on how to deal with some of the psychological issues raised in the 30-Day Plan, I express heartfelt thanks.

My family has rendered me unswerving support throughout the writing process: my brother and sister-in-law, Michael and Andee Shapiro, and my sister and brother-in-law, Marilyn and Michael McLaughlin. A daily presence during the writing of this UK edition of the book has been the memory of my parents, Eleanor DeWalt and Charles Shapiro.

The heroes and heroines of the book are the people you'll meet in its pages. The Chicago 7, members of the New York Police Department and several of the many New York City firefighters I've treated let me tell their stories in the book. I am grateful to them all. Like so many of my patients and readers, they are living proof that anyone can change his or her way of eating and lose considerable weight – even in 30 days. I applaud their success, and I am grateful to them for serving as inspiration to others.

Dr Howard M. Shapiro

OTHER RODALE BOOKS
AVAILABLE FROM PAN MACMILLAN

1-4050-3335-5	Picture Perfect Weight Loss	*Dr Howard M. Shapiro*	£14.99
1-4050-6715-2	The South Beach Diet Good Fats/Good Carbs Guide	*Dr Arthur Agatston*	£4.99
1-4050-6717-9	The South Beach Diet Cookbook	*Dr Arthur Agatston*	£20.00
1-4050-7732-8	How to Help Your Overweight Child	*Karen Sullivan*	£12.99
1-4050-7740-9	The Perfect Fit Diet	*Dr Lisa Sanders*	£12.99
1-4050-0666-8	Banish Your Belly, Butt & Thighs Forever!	*The Editors of* Prevention *Health Books for Women*	£10.99
1-4050-4099-8	Before the Heart Attacks	*Dr H. Robert Superko*	£10.99
1-4050-4179-X	Fit not Fat at 40+	Prevention *Health Books*	£12.99
1-4050-0665-X	Get a Real Food Life	*Janine Whiteson*	£12.99
1-4050-7741-7	The *Runner's World* Complete Book of Running for Beginners	*Amby Burfoot*	£16.99

All Pan Macmillan titles can be ordered from our website, *www.panmacmillan.com,* or from your local bookshop and are also available by post from:

Bookpost, PO Box 29, Douglas, Isle of Man IM99 1BQ
Credit cards accepted. For details:
Telephone: 01624 836000
Fax: 01624 670923
E-mail: bookshop@enterprise.net
www.bookpost.co.uk

Free postage and packing in the United Kingdom.

Prices shown above were correct at time of going to press.

Pan Macmillan reserve the right to show new retail prices on covers which may differ from those previously advertised in the text or elsewhere.

For information about buying *Rodale* titles in **Australia**, contact Pan Macmillan Australia. Tel: 1300 135 113; fax: 1300 135 103; e-mail: *customer.service@macmillan.com.au*; or visit: *www.panmacmillan.com.au*

For information about buying *Rodale* titles in **New Zealand**, contact Macmillan Publishers New Zealand Limited. Tel: (09) 414 0356; fax: (09) 414 0352; e-mail: *lyn@macmillan.co.nz*; or visit *www.macmillan.co.nz*

For information about buying *Rodale* titles in **South Africa**, contact Macmillan Publishers **South Africa**. Tel: (011) 325 5220; fax: (011) 325 5225; e-mail: *roshni@panmacmillan.co.za*